Boost your
Immune
system
naturally

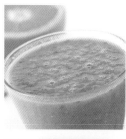

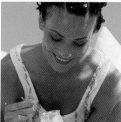

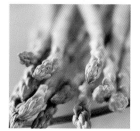

For Denis:

The Best Immune-System Booster A Girl Could Have

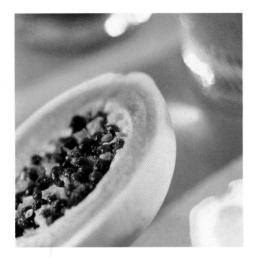

THIS IS A CARLTON BOOK

Design copyright © 2001 Carlton Books Limited
Text copyright © 2001 Beth MacEoin

This edition published in 2008
by Carlton Books Limited
20 Mortimer Street
London W1T 3JW

A CIP catalogue for this book is available
from the British Library.

ISBN 978 1 84732 047 6

Executive Editor: Sarah Larter
Editor: Janice Anderson
Art Editor: Adam Wright
Design: Zoë Mercer
Picture Research: Claire Gouldstone
Production: Garry Lewis
Jacket Design: Alison Tutton

Printed at Oriental Press, U.A.E.

Beth MacEoin

Boost your Immune system naturally

A lifestyle action plan

for strengthening your

natural defences

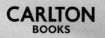

CARLTON
BOOKS

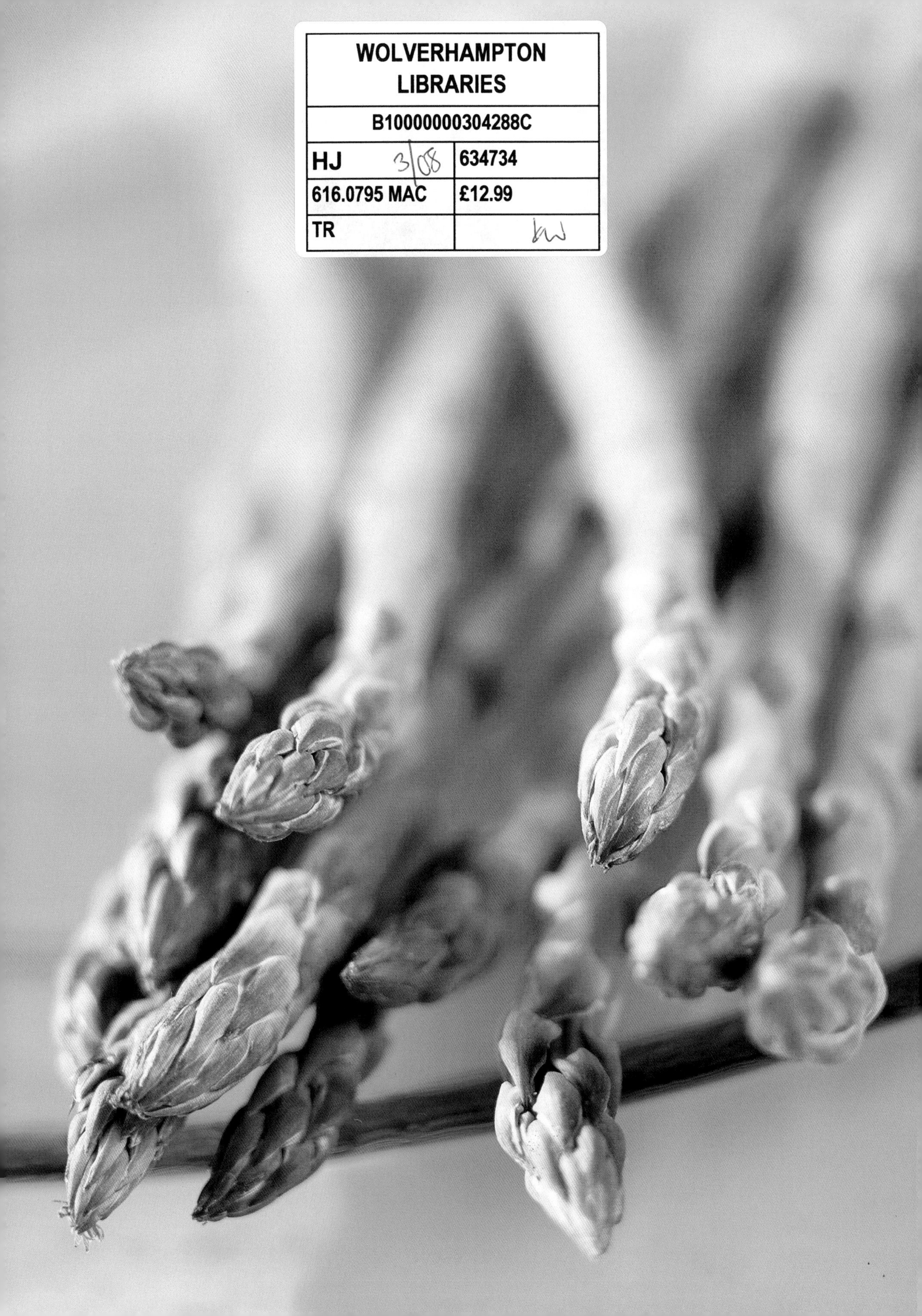

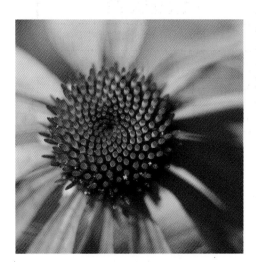

Introduction.........**6**

1
Self-Defence: How the Immune System Works.........**10**

2
Lifestyle Factors and Immunity.........**22**

3
Boosting Immunity through Nutrition.........**34**

4
Boosting Immunity with Antioxidants, Vitamins and Minerals.........**54**

5
Boosting Immunity with Natural Remedies.........**66**

6
Boosting Immunity with Exercise and Body-Conditioning Techniques.........**96**

7
Boosting Immunity with Relaxation.........**112**

Resources and Bibliography.........**124**

Index.........**126**

Contents

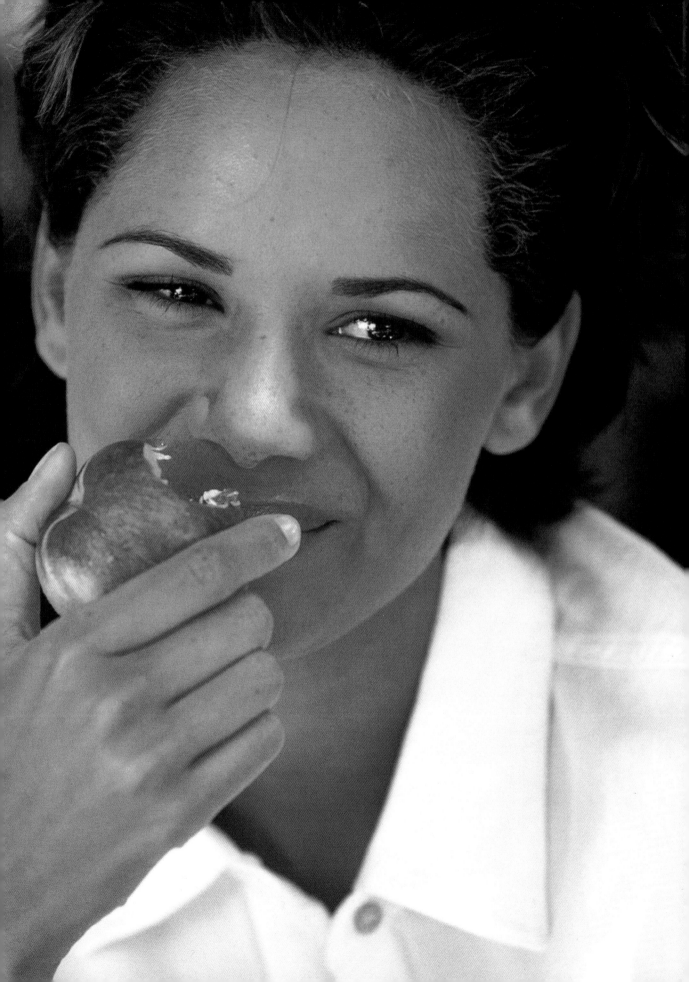

Without our body's immune system we can't survive. Although we are unaware of its working when we are in a state of good health, we are dependent on the effective functioning of its many components to fight the multiple foreign invaders that assault our bodies all the time.

The body is constantly coming into contact with bacteria and viruses that need to be dealt with effectively by the immune system. When it is working at peak efficiency we should not be conscious of any symptoms of ill health arising; at most, we may be aware of feeling slightly below par while the invader is being dealt with.

When we are generally in good health, if we go down with a cold, we may develop definite symptoms that last only a very short time – no more than three to five days. After that, we will generally make a full recovery without complications or an early recurrence of the problem. This sort of robust reaction would suggest that we have an immune system capable of fighting a cold virus vigorously and effectively: it is doing the job it was designed to do efficiently and decisively.

If, in contrast, we feel that we are constantly lurching from one infection to another, or seem to have a permanent cold all winter because we don't have the chance to recover from one bout before another moves in, the chances are that we have an immune system that is not coping well with the job that it is designed to do. Problems with the immune system have a generally compromising and limiting effect on the kind of health that we experience on all levels.

If the immune system is working in a balanced and effective way the benefits to us are impressively wide-ranging. Apart from being free of the strain of recurrent infections, we are also likely to find that we don't suffer from allergies, digestive problems, thrush, skin disorders or joint stiffness and pain. We should also discover that we enjoy optimum energy levels and an enhanced sense of well-being, which can have the added bonus of making us feel more emotionally balanced and resilient.

Well, we may ask, this sounds great, but how do we set about protecting and supporting the immune system? The answers to this question are in this book. It is a practical guide to the lifestyle factors that give a positive boost to the immune system, and to those that can compromise and deplete the functioning of the body's defence mechanisms.

Such guidance has become increasingly important in the modern world. Our bodies are constantly assaulted not only by invaders such as bacteria and viruses, but also by ever-increasing quantities of toxins from environmental pollution. Additional common factors known to put a strain on the immune system include physical and emotional stress, a poor diet deficient in the nutrients that boost the immune system, over-reliance on conventional medicines such as antibiotics for recurrent infections, and lack of exercise.

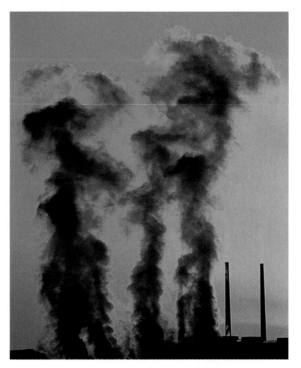

ABOVE: **Atmospheric pollution, such as is emitted by factory chimneys, puts extra strain on the immune system.**

Introduction

The good news is that we can turn this negative situation around by taking positive steps that have a tremendous effect in stimulating our own, in-built defence mechanisms. By taking the empowering steps of getting physically fitter, learning effective stress-reduction techniques, boosting our diets with powerful immune-system nutrients, and learning about appropriate use of nutritional supplements that help our bodies deal with environmental toxins, we can feel ourselves playing a major role in enabling our bodies to reach a state of optimum health.

In addition, we need to consider important developments in the growing field of alternative and complementary medicines. Unlike the conventional medical approach, which attempts to treat infections by using specific drugs that act as "magic bullets" targeted to eliminate specific bacteria, alternative therapies appear to work by strengthening the in-built capacity of the body to fight disease.

Alternative medicines are one of the greatest allies we can make use of if we want to boost our immune system. Natural approaches to healing such as traditional Chinese medicine, Western medical herbalism, homeopathy, or Ayurvedic medicine involve treatments that have no known side effects of the kind that are known to be associated with antibiotic use.

More significantly, alternative therapists view good health as being far more than mere absence of disease. Genuine health is seen as a positive entity in its own right that involves increased vitality, enhanced emotional well-being, freedom from the psychological and physical limitations of pain, and a basic confidence in the body's own capacity to fight infection.

Healthy immune system functioning is the cornerstone of positive health, and this book is dedicated to exploring the practical steps that can be taken to boost the body's own defences against lack-lustre health.

How this information is used is up to individual readers, since each one may come to this book from a different perspective. Some may feel they need a complete and fairly drastic overhaul because they experience a generally poor level of health and vitality on a day-to-day basis. For such people, a great deal will be gained by reading the book from cover to cover.

Others may feel they are generally fit, but are aware that they have specific problems, such as ones relating to their diet because it is made up mainly of "quick fix" foods. If there are specific areas like this that are causing problems, it may be enough to read the first two general chapters and the specific section that deals with the area of lifestyle that needs improvement.

Don't be afraid to use the information that follows as creatively as possible. Although the chapters have been written in a rational order, each chapter can stand as a self-sufficient unit. As a result, if there is a specific area that is of paramount interest to you, it's possible to go ahead and read it first if you really feel you don't want to wait. However you approach this book, I hope that you find your journey to an enhanced immune system performance is an exciting, exhilarating and enjoyable one.

TOP: **The drugs of conventional medicine act as "magic bullets" aimed at ridding the body of specific bacteria.**

OPPOSITE: **Alternative medicines, such as traditional Chinese medicine, aim to boost the body's capacity to heal itself.**

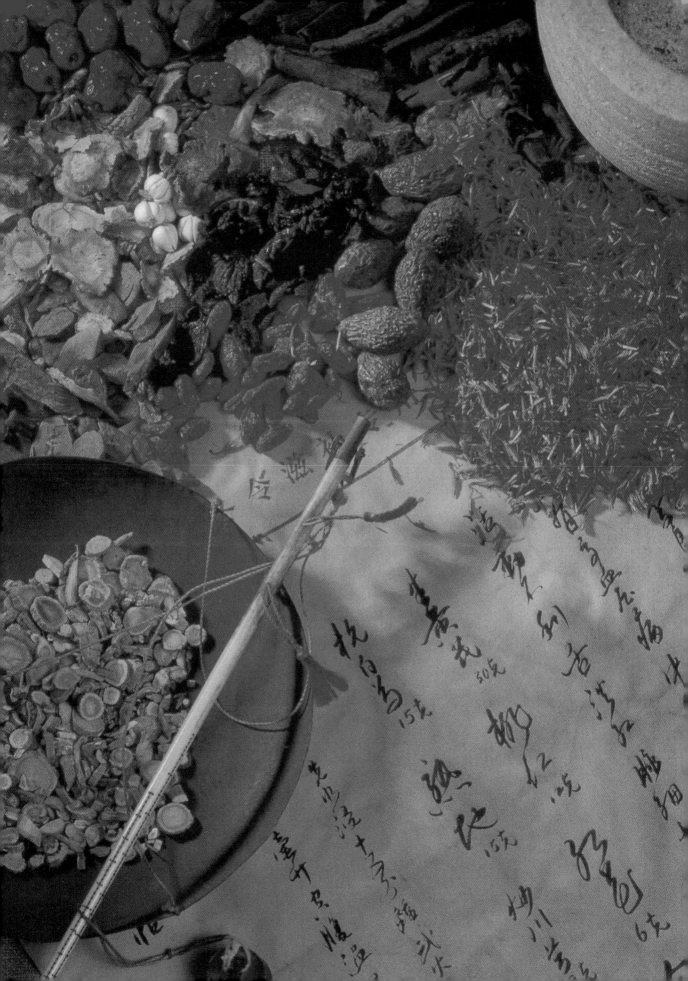

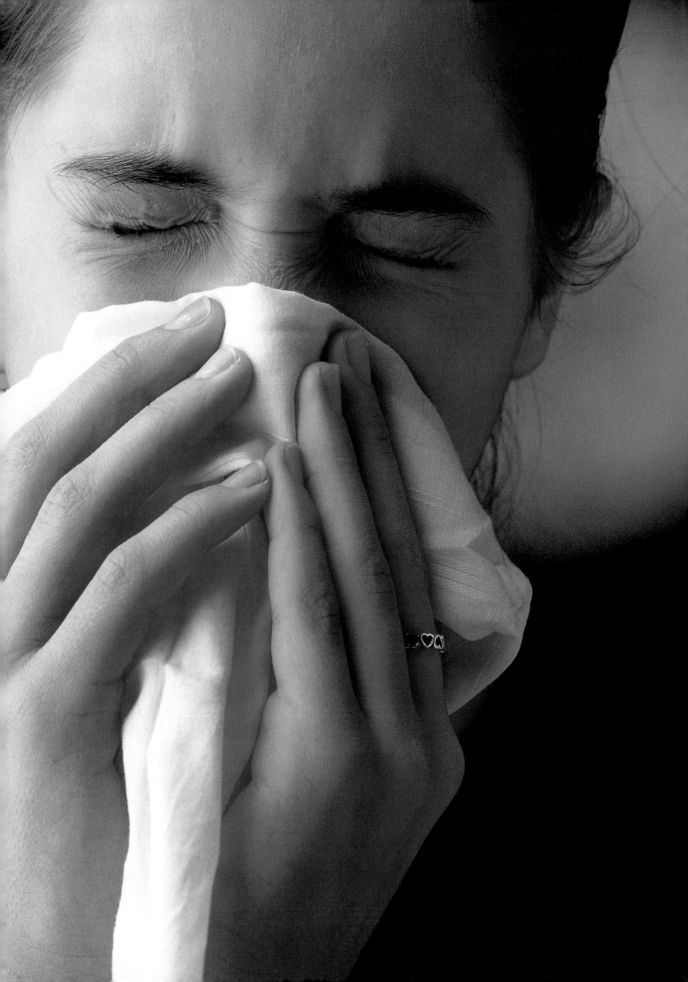

When we consider the intricacies and complexities of the immune system, it seems nothing short of miraculous that it does its job most of the time without any obvious problems occurring.

The immune system is astonishingly complicated, with links formed with every system of the body. It is made up of a complex network of organs that include the thymus gland, spleen, bone marrow, adenoids, tonsils, and the lymphatic system. Peak efficient working of the immune system depends on specialized cells called lymphocytes being formed in the bone marrow and thymus gland, and blood protein molecules called antibodies. There is also a complex series of checks and balances involving all the organs.

When these processes continue in a balanced way we enjoy optimum health and immunity to disease. If there is a continuing malfunction in the system, we are likely to lurch from one episode of illness to another, until our defences are able to re-balance themselves. If problems with our immune system continue long-term, we run the risk of moving from minor health problems such as allergies, recurrent infections, or skin disorders to more serious ones including auto-immune diseases such as rheumatoid arthritis and potentially fatal diseases such as various forms of cancer. Thankfully, new information about the important steps that can be taken to reduce vulnerability to such major diseases is being uncovered all the time.

Before you can take any steps to protect the strength and resilience of your immune system, it is important to learn something of how the body's defences work, so that you gain a better understanding of what you are attempting to do by taking immune-boosting measures. After all, it's very difficult to know how to solve a problem if the underlying causes of it are not understood.

What follows is not a detailed, cell-by-cell account of the structure and working of the body's immune system. Rather, it is a thumbnail sketch of the processes that are involved: once you understand the basic theory you'll be able to explore natural, practical measures to boost your health and vitality.

A Bird's Eye View of the Immune System

The immune system is made up of specialized cells that act as "search and destroy" agents, neutralizing the harmful effects of undesirable invaders such as bacteria, viruses and fungal and parasitic infections.

It is extremely important to understand that the immune system is not a separate entity in the body, but depends on a superbly orchestrated response on the part of a number of organs. The thymus gland, spleen, and bone

1 Self-Defence:
How The Immune System Works

marrow are influenced by the nervous system, and immune cells also carry receptors for brain hormones and transmitters. As a result, the state of a person's mental and emotional health can have a significant bearing on the working of the immune system.

First-line Immunity

We are born with an innate immunity, called natural, passive, or first-line immunity. This immunity is partly physical, beginning with the skin, which remains throughout our lives as our first barrier against infection. Babies are also born with substances in the body that destroy microorganisms. This basic level of early immunity can be further boosted if a baby is breast-fed, since breast-feeding allows antibodies to be passed on to the baby through the mother's milk.

BELOW: **Breast-fed babies acquire extra protection from antibodies passed to them in their mothers' milk.**

Second-line Immunity

This is the body's "adaptive immune system", often also referred to as "acquired immunity", since it involves a response to specific microbial invaders that may be encountered over the years. Once the body has developed an immunity to these specific organisms, it remains in the "memory" of the immune system so that if we should come in contact with that microbe on another occasion, a vigorous immune-system response can be switched on to deal with the invader in double-quick time.

Not only are the various components of the immune system capable of identifying infective agents that they may have been exposed to in the past, they are also capable of adopting a flexible approach so that they can accommodate aggressive attacks against an impressive array of new potential invading organisms.

The immune system mounts an individualized response to each micro-organism as it turns up. As a result, we may have

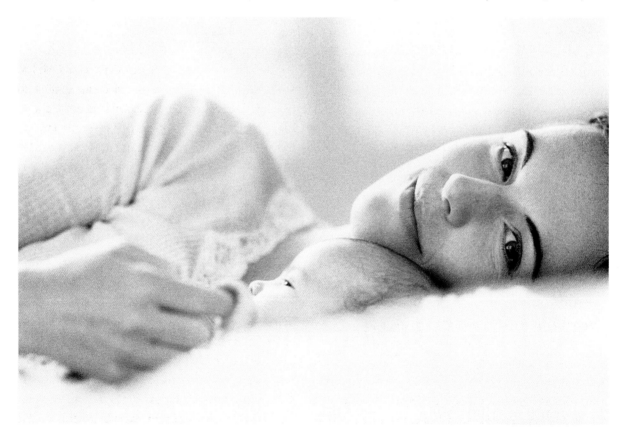

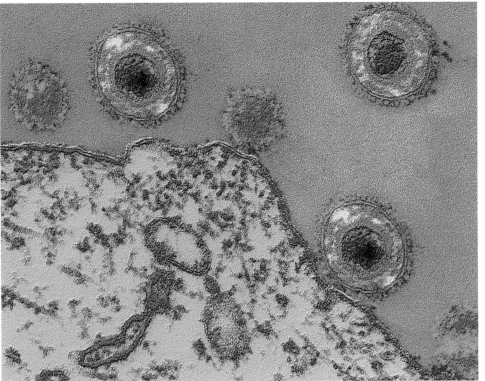

LEFT: **Exposure to the chicken pox virus (shown magnified here) demands a specialized response from the immune system.**

developed, as a result of getting measles, a natural immunity to the measles virus, but this will not help us fight chicken pox should the particular virus for that disease reach us. Our immune system must make a specific response to deal with that specific invader.

Vaccine-induced Immunity

Conventional medicine regards the process of vaccination as providing us with an effective defence against infectious diseases. However, as many alternative therapists have pointed out, the effects of vaccination may be subtly different from the strengthening effects on the immune system of naturally acquired immunity.

When we are exposed to a naturally occurring infection it usually enters our body through our first lines of defence, including the mucous membranes of the nose, mouth, throat, and vagina, which act as buffers so that the negative impact of microbes on the bloodstream can be reduced. With a naturally induced immune reaction, only a comparatively small amount of infective material makes its way beyond this first line of defence further into the body, where there is likely to be a vigorous response to it, though not so excessive a reaction that it results in its overall resistance being overwhelmed. On its way in, the invader will also come into contact with the tonsils, adenoids, and lymph nodes before entering the blood stream. As a result of this cumulative response, the invading agent brushes shoulders with the liver, spleen, thymus gland and bone marrow – all these before we become aware of any symptoms of invasion. This gives the optimum chance for effective mobilization of the immune system to occur.

When we are exposed to an artificially induced immune response such as a vaccine, a parallel, but significantly different reaction is set in motion. This is because modern vaccines involve comparatively large amounts of antigens which are injected directly into the bloodstream, effectively by-passing the body's first-line defences. As a result, the immune system registers this invasion as excessively traumatic and stressful. Alternative therapists regard this overly taxing assault on the immune system as being partly responsible for the way in which some patients will report that they have never felt fully well since a course of vaccinations. This can be especially the case if they felt that they were at a rather low ebb in the period just leading up to vaccination.

Additional problems that can emerge after a severe reaction to vaccination include allergies, persistent catarrhal problems, increased problems with asthma, and recurrent chest or ear infections.

The Immune System in Action

The very first barrier the body has against infection is the skin. Although many of us are most concerned about the quality of our skin from a cosmetic point of view, we should never forget that it plays a pivotal role in maintaining our overall health. This basic covering is designed to give an external structure to the body by holding things in (blood, muscles, and vital organs), but it also plays a central role in keeping undesirable visitors out.

Consider what happens if there is a break in the surface of the skin. Once this vitally important seal has been broken by a cut, scratch, or abrasion, the scene is set for outside invaders to get in and set up the process of infection. It therefore makes good sense to put effort into keeping the skin as supple and in as healthy a condition as possible. By doing so we are giving ourselves the best chance of keeping surface infection at bay.

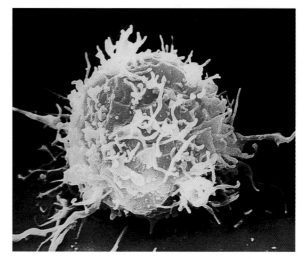

ABOVE: **T-lymphocytes have the ability to influence all tissues of the body as they move through the bloodstream.**

T-cells in Action

When the immune system mounts a response against an undesirable invader, the thymus gland produces specialized cells called T-cells. There appear to be four different kinds of immune system cells that are programmed by the thymus gland before birth. These are:

- Inducer T-cells, which are the first to identify that something foreign has been found which needs to be eliminated.
- Killer T-cells, whose job is to kill off alien proteins.
- Specialized cells called macrophages, which surround and absorb antigens.
- Suppressor T-cells, which call a halt to the attack when the invader has been dealt with.

T-cells are collectively called lymphocytes, which are a form of white blood cell that can be manufactured in the bone marrow, lymph nodes, liver, and the thymus gland. They have the potential to influence all body tissues as they travel through the lymphatic fluid and the bloodstream.

In addition, B-cells, formed by the bone marrow, act in tandem with the T-cells. These specialized cells are also lymphocytes, producing antibodies that are designed to eliminate and destroy threatening organisms when they are prompted to do so by helper T-cells. B-lymphocytes are the cells that hold the "memory" of any previous battle against an antigen. They are produced in the bone marrow and can act extremely swiftly when they recognize an invading antigen that they have encountered before.

This process of elimination stops when suppressor T-cells tell helper T-cells and B-cells to switch off the aggressive response. In addition, there are the killer T-cells, which are designed to kill off tumours and viruses.

When the immune system is in optimum shape, a very rapid attack can be set in motion against any organism that is recognized from the past. However, if the organism is a new visitor so that the immune system doesn't recognize it, it can take a few days for an effective attack to be set in motion. During this interval we may notice that our glands are painful, inflamed, and swollen – signs that the white blood cells are incubating a supply of antibodies in the lymph nodes, found in the neck, armpits, and groin.

When the body encounters an injury or infection it also manufactures white blood cells called macrophages, the job of which is to act as refuse collectors and scavengers, devouring

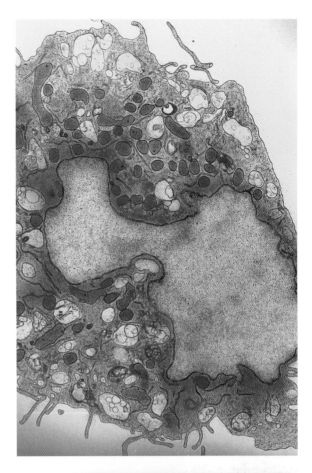

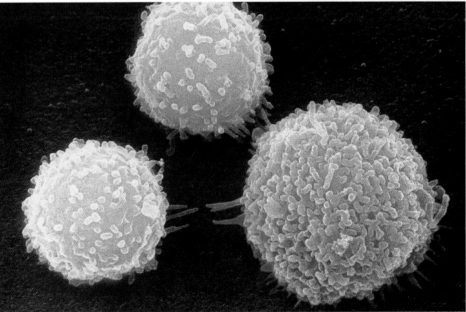

ABOVE RIGHT:
Macrophages work as the immune system's disposal unit, gobbling up unwanted debris on their way.

RIGHT: **An electron micrograph image of a macrophage (the blue cell) and two lymphocyte cells.**

and disposing of microbes and debris that are unfortunate enough to get in their way. Macrophages also produce a hormone called Interleukin 1, which is responsible for the characteristic rise in temperature that so often occurs when we are fighting an infection. The hormone Interleukin 2 also plays an important role in stimulating the action of killer T-cells.

It is the job of the immune system to react swiftly and decisively in eliminating any invader that is perceived to be a threat to our basic state of equilibrium and well-being. Whenever the latter is seen to be at risk, additional white blood cells are released from storage in the tonsils, thymus gland, spleen, and lymph glands.

It is important to bear in mind that the immune system is not just affected by threatening viruses, bacteria or toxins; it has also been shown to be profoundly influenced by severe physical and emotional shock, as well as by protracted stress.

Why We Need to Boost Our Self-defences

It has become very hard to ignore the problems that have been set in motion by an over-reliance on conventional drugs to fight our battles for us. Most of us will be aware of the difficulties that have emerged with antibiotic-resistant strains of bacteria that have become immune to treatment with antibiotics. This can make us feel anxious and vulnerable when we realize that we can no longer depend on conventional drugs alone to solve our health problems for us.

However, we are free to take positive steps towards boosting our own immunity so that we are unlikely to need conventional drugs to sort out every minor infection. Used appropriately, these measures can also give the added bonus

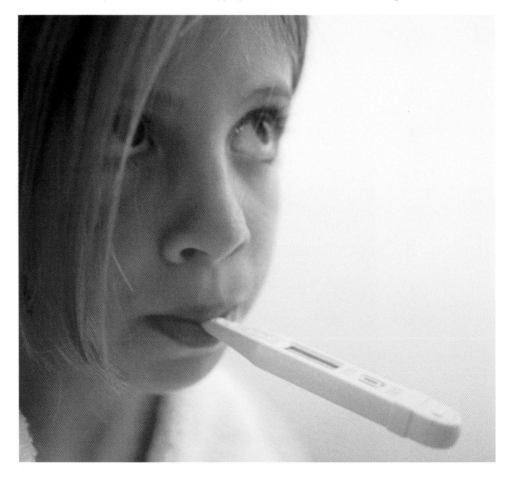

RIGHT: **A moderately high temperature can be a sign that the immune system is working effectively.**

of greater clarity of mind, enhanced emotional balance, greater energy levels, and a much greater confidence in our own bodies.

It has become clear that it can be positively undesirable and counter-productive to undermine immune-system performance by intervening with conventional drugs on a routine or too early basis. Take as a basic example a dose of flu: the best thing we can do to help ourselves through this illness without troublesome complications is to concentrate on the practical measures that will give the immune system the support it needs.

These include rest above all else, since a great deal of energy is needed to fight infection, without diverting it elsewhere. Not only does being up and about make our own situation worse, but it also has the counter-productive effect of spreading the illness to others. Fever is best kept down by taking lots of fluids and avoiding heavy meals, rather than relying too much on painkillers in order to keep going.

Most conventional drugs work by dampening down the response that the body makes to get rid of infection. For instance, a moderately high temperature is a sign of the immune system working in a highly effective way. If this response is suppressed by taking painkillers, it is more likely that we will take longer to get over the infection.

The same is true of using medication designed to temporarily suppress a cough or dry up mucus discharges from the nasal passages. The reason why the body produces a cough or a streaming nose is to get as much toxic waste out as fast as possible so that recovery will be in double quick time. If the process is interfered with, we can be pretty sure that we are going to feel unwell for longer than we would if we supported the body's capacity for self-healing.

Of course, we must also use our common sense and recognize the difference between a serious, life-threatening infection and a minor, acute problem where we have the time to support our bodies safely through to recovery. In practice, this is not so difficult. We know that minor problems such as acute coughs, colds, and stomach upsets can be dealt with by sensible self-help measures, and that serious illnesses such as meningitis, pneumonia, and bronchitis (especially in those with a history of asthma or in the elderly) need swift conventional medical treatment, usually involving appropriate drugs and practical measures such as rehydration, in order to give the patient the best chance of making a full recovery.

How our Health can be Affected by Reduced Immunity

Potential health problems that can surface as a consequence of compromised immune-system performance can be wide-ranging in their nature and severity, from skin problems that are minor annoyances to life-threatening diseases. They can include any of the following:

Feeling Generally "Run Down" or Under Par

This is one of the most common problems encountered by alternative therapists. Many patients seek treatment with alternative medicines because they feel they just are not as well as they should be. Very often, tests for possible causes have been done (such as checking for glandular fever, anaemia or problems with thyroid gland functioning), only for them to come up with negative results.

Common problems that can arise as a result of a generally sluggish or poorly functioning immune system include recurrent colds, repeated bouts of urinary tract infections, generally poor resistance to any bug that happens to be doing the rounds, and a general sense of exhaustion and weariness. The latter can have a knock-on effect on the emotional equilibrium and general sense of well-being, since many people begin to feel anxious and depressed if they are constantly aware that they are not meeting the demands of day-to-day living.

Hypersensitivities and Allergies

If the body's immune system becomes hypersensitive, it can go into overdrive and over-react to agents that are under normal conditions are relatively harmless. Such innocuous substances as pollen, animal fur, house dust, fungal spores

BELOW: **Animal fur, including the long, easily shed hair of cats, is a common trigger of an allergic response.**

RIGHT: **Nuts are another cause of allergic reactions; peanuts, in particular, can cause – fortunately, in only a very few cases – severe anaphylactic shock.**

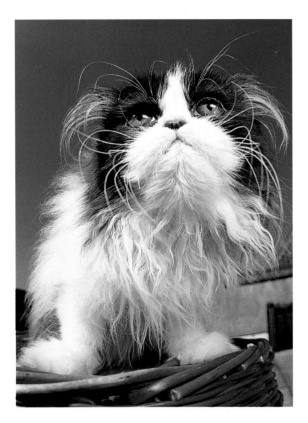

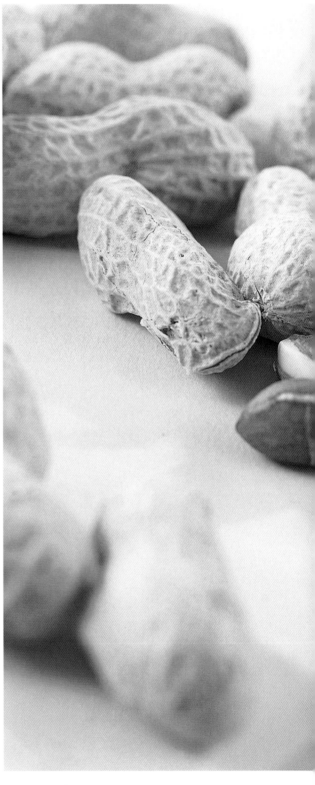

and certain foods, including peanuts, fish, and shellfish can all cause such reactions. These, in turn, can lead to bouts of hay fever, asthma, eczema, and severe food allergies.

There are two different types of allergic response, classed as IgE or cell-mediated. A classic allergic response is characterized by a rise of IgE antibodies (protective soluble proteins manufactured by B-lymphocyte cells) that trigger an immune-system reaction causing an inflammatory response. As an IgE antibody comes across an invader, it triggers a release of chemicals, including histamine. This is why a common conventional medical solution to allergic symptoms involves prescribing antihistamines in an effort to dampen down or lessen the allergic response.

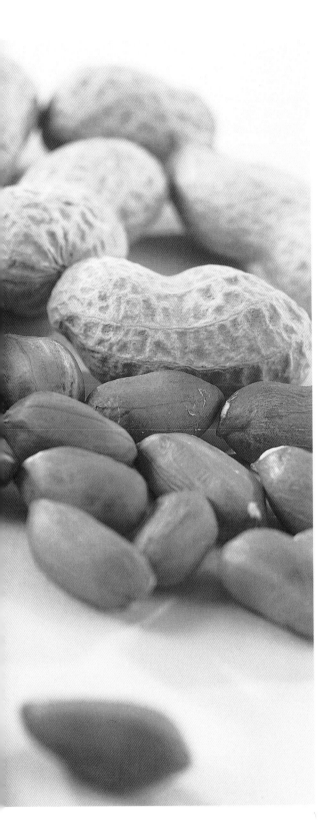

An IgE reaction is swift in nature and easily defined. A cell-mediated response may result in more subtle symptoms that do not surface rapidly and can include anything from digestive disorders such as irritable bowel syndrome to hyperactivity and poor concentration in children. Symptoms may be sparked off by exposure to a range of everyday foods including sugar, tea, coffee, wheat, corn and eggs.

Since an IgE allergic response can be identified through a blood test but a cell-mediated response cannot, there is a tendency on the part of the orthodox medical profession to suggest that food intolerances aren't causing an allergic response. This can be very frustrating for people who are sure they have a negative reaction to certain specific foods.

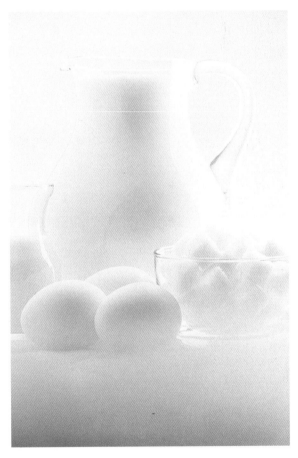

ABOVE: **Eggs and dairy foods made from cow's milk, as well as the milk itself, are all recognized triggers of allergic reactions.**

Auto-immune Disorders

If helper T-cells become too enthusiastic in doing their job of attacking invaders, they can make the mistake of turning against the body's own tissues. This problem occurs because the immune system can no longer differentiate between a threatening invader and harmless cells, with resulting periodic symptoms of inflammation and pain. Chronic health problems that arise as a consequence of skewed auto-immune responses include rheumatoid arthritis, corneal ulcers, and multiple sclerosis.

AIDS and HIV

As we have seen, a healthily-functioning immune system depends on helper and suppressor T-cells working in harmony, so that the appropriate antibodies are in optimum supply to protect the body. A serious problem can develop if the suppressor cells become dominant, resulting in the immune system becoming weakened or deficient. This can occur as a result of a genetically inherited condition or when an opportunistic infection, such as the HIV virus, moves in. HIV works by attacking helper T-cells, so that an essential link in the functioning of the immune system is lost. The result is a cycle of recurrent infections, including chronically swollen glands, thrush, cold sores, genital herpes and extreme weariness and exhaustion.

Cancer

"Cancer" is a collective term that covers approximately 500 different diseases. A diagnosis of cancer is instinctively dreaded by any unwell person. However, it should be understood that cancer can manifest itself in many different ways and in varying degrees of severity and seriousness, depending on many factors.

The outcome of a cancer diagnosis can vary enormously,

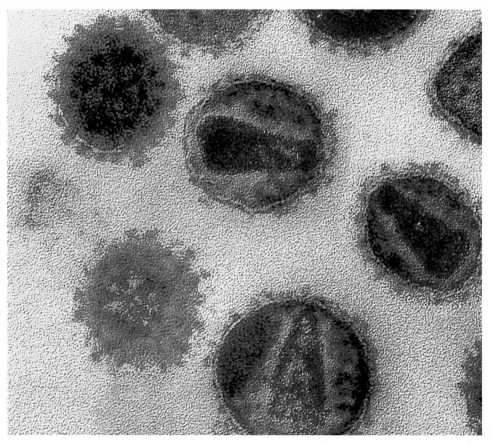

LEFT: **A well-balanced, efficient immune system response requires helper and suppressor T-cells to work in tandem; if they do not, we may become vulnerable to opportunistic infections such as HIV, the virus pictured here.**

depending on how quickly the diagnosis is made, where the cancer is located, and on more general aspects such as inherited factors and quality of lifestyle. In fact, the immune system regularly eliminates potentially cancerous cells as they are produced. Cancer occurs when abnormal cells multiply in the bodies at such a rate that the immune system cannot control them.

Normal cell division goes on all the time in the body. Sometimes a dividing cell is produced that has failed to be correctly genetically coded. If this mutant cell is left free to multiply rapidly it has a strong chance of developing into a cancer. If we are in good health and our immune system is working efficiently, our bodies have the potential to deal with such potentially cancerous cells. On the other hand, mutant cells have an elusive and resilient quality, sometimes developing a surface protective barrier in order to try to evade destruction by killer T-cells.

Several factors have been identified as influencing the risk of being vulnerable to developing cancer. They include:

GENETIC INHERITANCE
If women have close female relatives (mother, sisters, or aunts) who have suffered from breast cancer they are four time more likely than an average woman to be vulnerable to this cancer.

LIFESTYLE
Genetic inheritance cannot be altered, but positive changes can be made to lifestyle, eliminating as many as possible of the negative aspects that can leave us more vulnerable to developing serious illness. Basic protective measures include:
- Cutting down alcohol intake.
- Giving up smoking and avoiding passive smoking wherever possible.
- Cutting down on intakes of dietary fats such as margarine, butter, cheese and cream.
- Avoiding exposure to radiation or too much sunbathing (especially without adequate protection).
- Avoiding contact with certain chemicals such as the benzopyrenes used in dry cleaning.

EMOTIONAL WELL-BEING
Our emotions can play a significant role in promoting optimum immune-system functioning or undermining the body's defences. Emotions that appear to play a powerful negative role in suppressing health and vitality include repressed anger, unexpressed grief and protracted depression. This appears to be due to the way in which extended psychological stress and unopposed negative emotions lead to a depressed functioning of the immune system, while positive, pleasurable experiences appear to do the reverse. So now it's official: uplifting, pleasurable experiences are good for our health!

Now we have examined the negative side of the problems that can occur as a result of glitches in the functioning of the immune system, it is time to move on to considering the practical steps that may be taken to boost natural self-defences. In the next chapter, the fundamental lifestyle factors necessary to maximize immunity levels, well-being and vitality are examined.

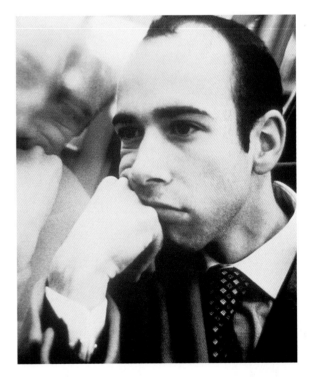

ABOVE: **Our emotional health plays a key role in supporting or undermining the functioning of the immune system.**

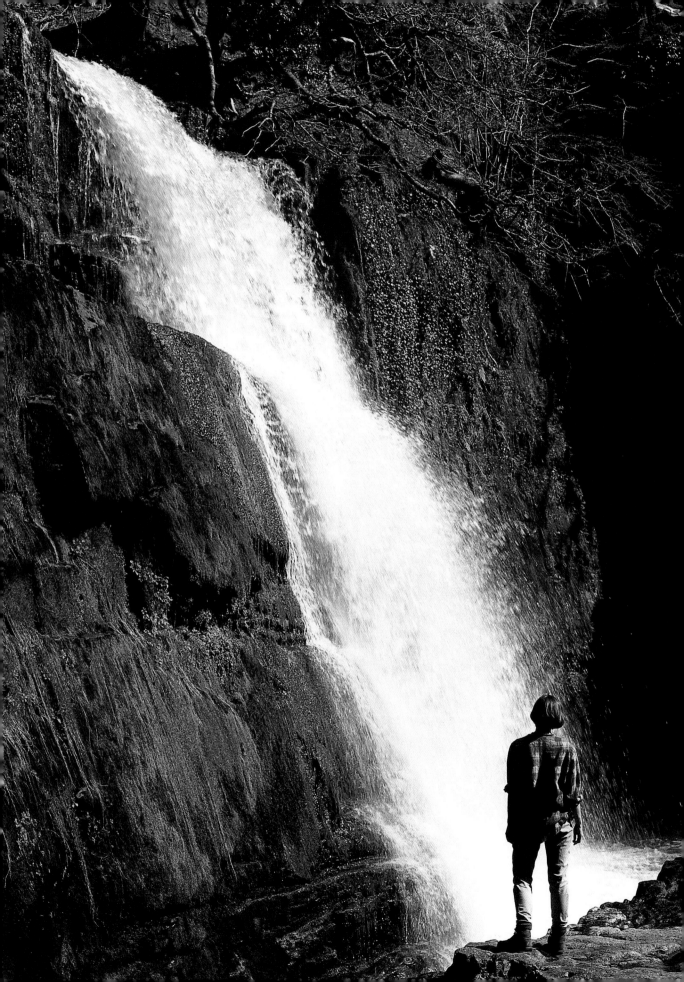

This chapter gives a general overview of the basic issues you need to consider if you want to adopt the lifestyle changes that are going to boost your capacity for self-healing. It is deliberately approached in the style of a quick tour, delivering the basic information as concisely as possible. A more expanded practical approach to each major topic – nutrition, exercise, and emotional well-being – is given in the chapters that follow.

Taking Charge

It is a wonderful thing when you come to realize that instead of resigning yourself to experiencing a lacklustre kind of health every day, there are simple steps to take that will positively revolutionize how you feel mentally, emotionally, and physically.

Of course, everyone has to work within the boundaries of certain basic realities, including the fact that the body's immune system does not function as decisively or efficiently as we get older. This appears to be linked to the way in which the thymus gland slowly shrinks as the body ages, resulting in a reduced potential for effective immunity. The process involves the production of a hormone called thymulin secreted by the thymus which triggers a reduction in the production of T-cells. As a result, the B-cells which work in tandem with the T-cells are unable to produce antibodies,

which can leave you more vulnerable to recurrent infections. Energy levels and sleep patterns are also likely to change as the body reacts to the ageing process.

There is no need to accept any of this with a resigned sense of inevitability – a very dangerous approach. Once someone adopts the belief that there is little point in making positive changes in the quality of their life because they are bound to get old and experience declining health, they are ensuring that they will feel under par most of the time.

There is also a good chance that people with such an attitude will be at risk of visible signs of premature ageing, and may also develop the symptoms of degenerative diseases such as circulatory problems or arthritis well before they need to. Following this passive path is also almost guaranteed to induce a feeling of physical weariness, as well as an emotional and mental lack of sparkle. This has a knock-on effect of lowering self-esteem, which can make you less sociable, which in turn makes you feel more unpopular and depressed ... and so the negative cycle gathers momentum.

Let's not forget, however, that in the same way that a negative cycle can gather momentum, so the destructive trend can be effectively reversed, by putting positive lifestyle measures in place. While it remains necessary to work within realistic boundaries, acknowledging that the immune system won't function in the same way at fifty as it did at fifteen, it is still possible to support the body to fight infection as

Lifestyle 2 factors and Immunity

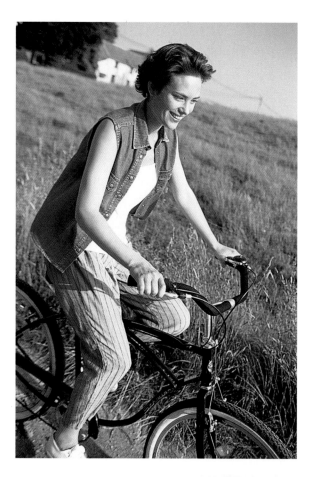

effectively as possible, while also boosting energy levels and encouraging maximum emotional and mental balance.

There are several starting points from which to set a positive cycle of change in motion. You may start with improving your diet, taking up an enjoyable system of exercise, or consulting an alternative practitioner. Once energy levels have been given an initial boost from any of these important changes, you are likely to find you have more enthusiasm and commitment to make further improvements. These could include finding out about relevant nutritional supplements, or using alternative remedies at home in order to deal with minor ailments.

This is likely to give a greater sense of working in harmony with the body as it comes to feel stronger and healthier. Subsequently it will boost levels of confidence and self-esteem. These are the catalysts that are often needed to give the final push towards sorting out issues that may have been put on hold for too long and may involve making positive changes or improvements with regard to jobs, social life or close relationships.

The foundation of this sense of body confidence lies in boosting the immune system effectively. After all, how is it possible to feel vibrant and positive if you can't feel confident

ABOVE: **Exercise plays a key role in promoting physical, emotional and mental balance.**

RIGHT: **Pleasurable, positive and uplifting experiences have been shown to play significant roles in supporting good health.**

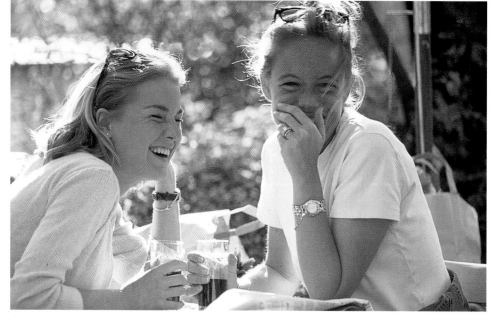

about enjoying high-level health? Once you know you can depend on your body not to let you down, or more importantly, discover the practical, trouble-shooting measures that can be used when a minor crisis does occur, your whole perspective on reaching your potential for optimum health will take a massive turn towards the positive.

The Basic Self-Defence Plan

Four important lifestyle factors, known to affect overall immune-system performance, form the basis of a good self-defence plan for the immune system. They are:

- The mind/body link with immunity, emphasizing the importance of effective stress-reduction techniques and positive thinking.
- Basic body care from within, with an emphasis on the importance of good nutrition.
- Basic body conditioning, including exercise, hydrotherapy and de-toxing skin brushing techniques.
- Radical self-defence for the whole system, via alternative and complementary medicine.

Each of these is introduced here before being given a whole chapter for detailed discussion later.

The Mind/Body Link and Immunity

Very few of us are unaware of the negative impact that excessive stress levels can have on our overall health. Doctors practising conventional medicine acknowledge that a large number of conditions can be triggered, or aggravated, by excessive physical, mental, or emotional stress. These health problems include irritable bowel syndrome, tension headaches, migraines and skin conditions such as eczema and psoriasis that appear to respond negatively to emotional stress.

In the relatively new field of psychoneuroimmunology, increasingly important links are being discovered between healthy mental and emotional balance and positive immune-system functioning, suggesting that the way in which we think and react emotionally on a day-to-day basis can have a profound effect on the functioning of the immune system and the average quality of health enjoyed on all levels.

Studies at New York's Mount Sinai Hospital School of Medicine in the late 1970s showed that the functioning of the immune system could be depressed following bereavement, protracted grieving or depression. Other problems that appeared to be linked to emotional stress included a higher risk of developing hardening of the arteries, high blood pressure and on-going digestive problems.

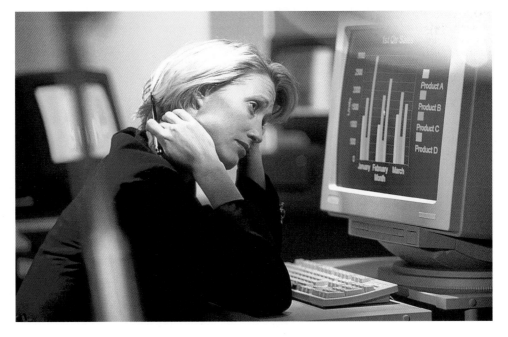

RIGHT: **Negative stress, such as tiredness caused by overwork, can be responsible for a range of chronic health problems.**

Specific links between the mind and the immune system were revealed by a more recent study carried out at the University of Reading in England. Participants in the study who deliberately induced positive memories had elevated immune antibodies when their saliva samples were tested before and after recalling the pleasurable memory. In contrast, those who deliberately brought to mind unhappy or guilt-ridden memories were shown to have depressed antibody levels.

When people become aware of the negative impact of stressful experiences on overall immunity, perhaps by noticing a commonly-occurring pattern in response to those pressures, something that previously may have been rather inexplicable begins to make sense. It is quite a common occurrence for people to struggle through the challenge of physical, emotional and mental stress, only to collapse with an acute illness once things have begun to relax a little. This can take the form of a bout of 'flu, a heavy cold, migraine or a severe digestive upset that leaves the sufferer exhausted and immobile.

There is an internal logic to this process. When we are exposed to maximum stress levels and these continue unabated for too long, our general resistance is undermined. The body appears to have an extraordinary coping mechanism that allows a person under stress to continue to function while the stress is at its height, almost as though the body knows that collapsing at this stage would be a total disaster. It continues to function, while it is in fact "running on empty", using up energy reserves and surviving on adrenaline as much as anything else.

Once the immediately stressful phase has been dealt with and things begin to calm down, comes the most likely moment for the body to choose to temporarily give up. This is why migraine sufferers will almost certainly develop a migraine once a deadline has been met, during a weekend or during the holidays: in other words, when taking it easy will not cause massive disruption. Developing an acute problem that forces us to spend some time in bed is how the body often ensures that we overcome the aftermath of stress.

If this happens as a one-off episode on a very infrequent basis, it can be dealt with. If, on the other hand, it becomes a repeating pattern of illness that is never quite recovered from, the sufferer must take the issue of stress reduction techniques seriously. This is essential if the situation is to be turned around in order to experience genuinely positive health.

Practical advice on stress-banishing techniques and how to avoid negative thought patterns can be found in Chapter 6, "Boosting Immunity With Relaxation" (page 96).

The "weekend" or "holiday" migraine is a sure sign of an overload of stress.

Basic Body Care from Within: Nutrition

Very few of us can be unaware by now of the profound importance of the quality of the food we eat on a regular basis if we want to enjoy an on-going sense of well-being and vitality. Trite as it may sound, we really "are what we eat". Our diet provides the basic material that the body depends upon for such basic functions as energy and heat production, and the building, maintenance and repair of body tissues.

It stands to reason that if we put rubbish in, we are likely to get rubbish in return. It is a natural consequence that we will feel less than bouncing with health with a diet made up mainly of junk foods combined with regular smoking, excessive consumption of alcohol and regular intake of high-caffeine drinks such as coffee, strong tea and fizzy colas. Not only are all these seriously deficient in the basic nutrients that the body demands, but they also form the additional hazard of depleting the body of essential nutrients without putting anything valuable back.

If you make a point of including foods in your daily eating plan that have a reputation for immune-system boosting properties, you will be giving yourself the maximum opportunity for experiencing high-level health. Such a way of eating certainly need not involve a spartan, harsh or overly restrictive diet. Following a balanced approach, leading to a regained sense of pleasure from what you eat, is essential if you are to be truly well and healthy.

Adopting too faddy and restrictive an approach to eating can cause problems – different from the problems arising out of eating junk foods, but important issues, nevertheless. When taking on an eating plan designed to give the body's

ABOVE: **Junk foods should always be avoided when you are aiming for maximum health and vitality.**

capacity for immunity a maximum boost, it is important to aim for a well-balanced, varied diet that does not make you feel socially isolated or deprived. You should even discover that you enjoy what you eat even more than previously, because you will be feeling more aware and energized as a result of increased levels of vitality.

Details of how to eat well on a regular basis in order to boost the immune system are given in the following chapter, but here is a summary of the broad principles:

- Your basic diet should include as much fresh, raw fruit and vegetables as possible. Especially important ingredients include fruit and vegetables that are rich in antioxidant nutrients because these have a vitally important role in boosting the immune-system. Such foods are easy to spot because they are generally bright orange, red, dark green or yellow in colour.
- Opt for regular helpings of essential fatty acids (EFAs) which can be found in oily fish, certain cold-pressed virgin vegetable oils and nuts.
- Drink plenty of filtered or bottled spring water in order to flush out the system, improve skin quality and guard against toxic waste building up in the system as a result of constipation.
- Include lots of complete proteins from a vegetable source in the diet by combining pulses and beans with whole grains and cereals.
- Always choose wholegrain versions of rice, pasta and flour, avoiding white, refined products whenever possible.
- If dairy foods are a favourite have them as a treat rather than in large quantities on a daily basis.
- Always make a point of choosing organic, free-range produce whenever possible.

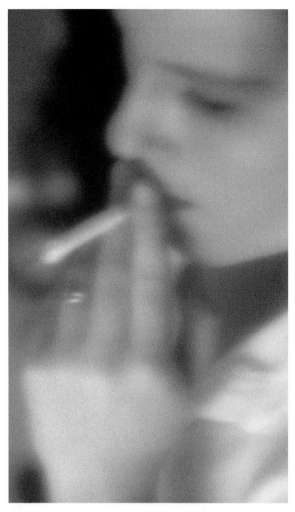

ABOVE: **Smoking is a major health hazard; it also contributes greatly to outward signs of premature ageing.**

- Avoid any foods that look as though they have been unduly processed and tampered with in order to prolong their shelf-life artificially. Major culprits include anything that has been dehydrated, canned, vacuum-packed or includes a bewildering array of preservatives and additives.
- Find alternatives to foods that contain a high proportion of refined white sugar. If fizzy drinks are a problem, try the many carbonated varieties made from unsweetened, natural fruit juices and sparkling mineral water instead. Some naturally produced cereal bars or organic, wholemeal biscuits flavoured with honey can satisfy a sweet tooth. Also look out for canned organic baked beans which do not have huge quantities of white sugar added to them.
- Watch alcohol, coffee and tea intake. See Chapter 3, "Boosting Immunity Through Nutrition" (page 34) for advice on how to set about this.
- Try to avoid smoking or passive smoking at all costs. You will find good advice on how to quit the habit in the next chapter, with an explanation of why this is a priority if you are concerned about protecting and boosting the immune system.

Basic Body Conditioning: Exercise, Hydrotherapy and De-toxing Skin Brushing Techniques

Taking regular aerobic exercise has a profound effect on overall health, especially when it is part of a fitness programme that includes additional exercise systems that encourage muscular stretching, flexibility, stamina and relaxation. Not only does this combination of physical activity have an impressively positive effect on physical stamina, body shape, energy levels and emotional well-being, but it is also an essential ingredient in any plan to boost your immune system.

This is because of the way that regular, low-impact exercise conditions the heart and lungs, enhancing your potential for making maximum use of the oxygen you inhale. In addition, such exercise also greatly stimulates the flow of lymphatic fluid, which plays a pivotal role in helping in the fight against infection.

Regular exercise also brings an important cosmetic benefit in the form of reducing cellulite production. A marked improvement in the severity and distribution of cellulite is an important clue as to how well the immune system is working. Details on managing and minimizing cellulite are in Chapter 6, "Boosting Immunity With Exercise" (page 96).

When selecting an exercise system it is absolutely essential to make sure that whatever activity is chosen is going to be enjoyable, and well suited to your individual tempera-

RIGHT: **Swimming is one of the most enjoyable ways of giving the heart and lungs a conditioning workout.**

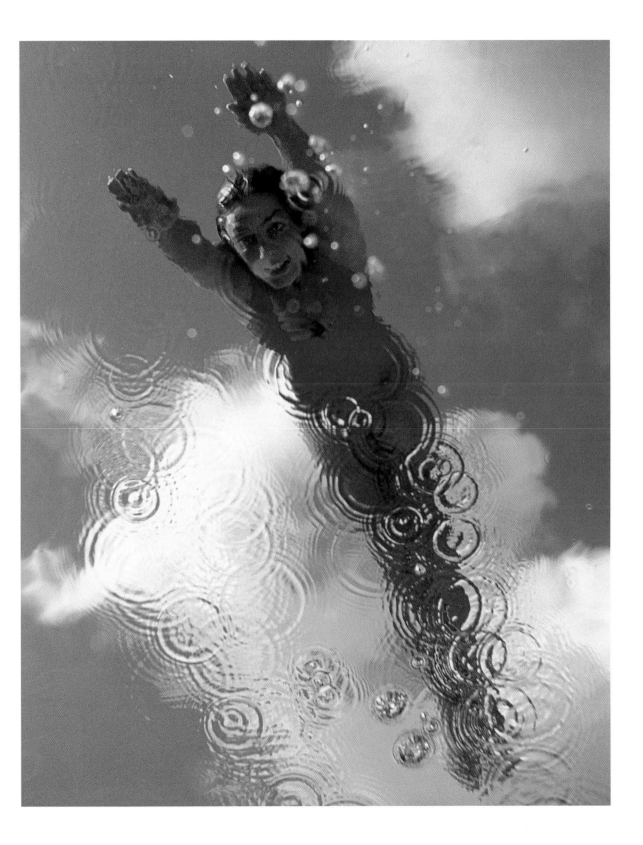

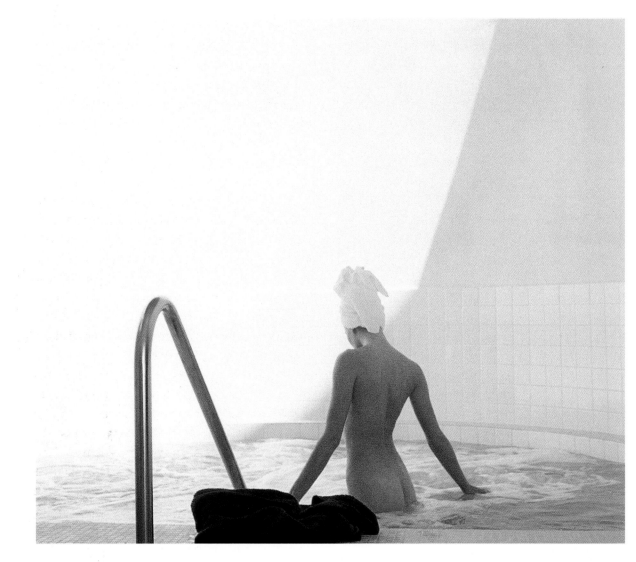

ABOVE: **Hydrotherapy stimulates the flow of lymphatic fluid, improving the performance of the immune-system and skin tone.**

ment. If it isn't, the plan is going to be doomed to failure. After all, who is going to stick relentlessly to a physical activity that they find mind-numbingly boring? There are so many exercise possibilities available that there is no need to feel pressured into doing something because it is considered beneficial. Always make sure the magic ingredients of pleasure and fun are also there. Possible options to consider include dancing, skiing, rowing, walking, power yoga, cycling, swimming or sports such as tennis, volleyball and badminton.

Whatever activities are chosen, they must be practical enough to fit into the way your week is structured so that a regular time can be set aside for them and the commitment to getting fit can be kept up. A regular routine is the secret to a successful fitness programme, since maximum benefit can be gained from relatively short sessions three or four times a week. This has a much more beneficial effect on overall health than doing nothing for a few weeks, and then trying to make up for lost time by frantically spending two or three hours at the gym. The latter approach is much more likely to end up in injury and exhaustion than in enhanced fitness.

You will find lots of good advice on putting together an appropriate exercise programme in Chapter 6.

Dry skin brushing techniques are also a valuable and "hands on" way of stimulating the efficient flow of lymphatic fluid through the body. Positive results of the techniques are that toxins are eliminated more effectively, nutrients are transported more efficiently to the tissues and the immune system benefits by working more smoothly and vigorously. There are specific details on how to set about dry skin brushing and hydrotherapy techniques that can be used at home in Chapter 6.

Radical Self-defence for the Whole System: Alternative and Complementary Medicine

Complete systems of healing such as Western medical herbalism, traditional Chinese medicine or homeopathy are aptly termed alternative medical systems, since they provide a radically alternative view of healing to the approach of conventional medicine.

Orthodox medical opinion often describes the functioning of the body in mechanistic terminology. The body can be seen as being made up of a complex series of superbly intricate, inter-dependent parts. When all is going well, the body appears to be a spectacularly impressive machine that has infinite scope for adapting to changing circumstances. However, malfunctions in this superb machinery can arise for a number of reasons and, if not rectified promptly, can lead to the emergence of signs and symptoms of ill health.

Common factors that interrupt the smooth working of the body can include specific infections, accidents and injuries, or physical demands such as excessive physical strain. In addition, the ageing process is seen from a conventional medical perspective as bringing with it associated problems of "wear and tear" that will surface in the form of symptoms related to inflammation and pain in joints and muscles.

Stress and unhealthy lifestyle factors such smoking, a poor-quality diet deficient in essential nutrients, or drinking excessive amounts of alcohol are also increasingly gaining recognition as factors that can cause glitches in the smooth working of the body's systems. The body has the capacity to adapt and cope with the toxic burdens imposed by a temporary unhealthy lifestyle, but will eventually become overwhelmed and begin to show signs of ill health if the pressure continues for too long. These may commonly take the form of persistently low energy levels, an inability to relax, poor sleep patterns and a whole host of digestive problems including indigestion, poor appetite or troublesome alternation between diarrhoea and constipation.

As an extension of this mechanistic approach to disease, the majority of conventional drug treatments focus on eliminating specific organisms, chemical imbalances or excessive inflammation from the body. Sadly, although these can seem nothing short of miraculous in their short-term action, well-documented problems have arisen in response to this "magic bullet" approach to treatment. These problems are linked to various undesirable side-effects that can emerge as a result of drug treatment, despite the fact that a great deal of time, effort and money is invested in trying to make these drugs as streamlined in their action as possible.

The groups of drugs where these problems are familiar include antibiotics, anti-inflammatories and steroids. Any of these kinds of drug has the potential for setting off a negative chain reaction where fresh symptoms can arise – for instance, digestive upsets in response to taking anti-inflammatories, or thrush following a course of antibiotics – which often require the prescription of additional drugs to eliminate the new symptoms.

Since these additional drugs also have the potential for setting up even more side-effects, we can see how easy it is to work out which symptoms are related to the original illness, and which are triggered by side-effects. The issue of side-effects becomes even more of a concern where powerful drugs such as oral steroids are being used, since these are known to have a powerfully depressing effect on the immune system.

The alternative approach to medical treatment is very different. Instead of concentrating on finding treatments that are targeted against specific bacteria or viruses, alternative therapists are more concerned with concentrating on what makes us susceptible to illness taking hold in the first place. For instance, many people know they only have to stand near someone who is sneezing for them to come down with a severe cold or sore throat. In such a situation, treatment from an alternative practitioner would concentrate on finding effective ways of supporting the body in fighting off infection more robustly and decisively.

Depending on the therapy that is chosen, the possible ways of strengthening the body are very varied indeed. They could include stimulating the body's natural resistance to infection by using specific herbal medicines, acupuncture treatments or individually chosen homeopathic medicines.

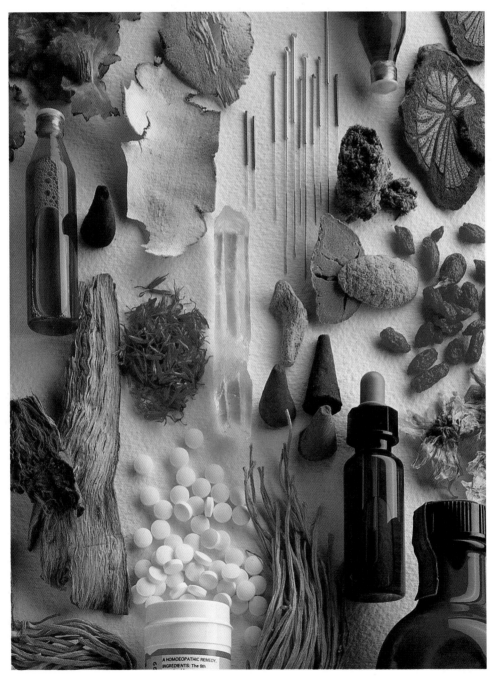

LEFT: **A selection of the great range of remedies used by alternative medicine therapists. Alternative medical treatment aims to restore the whole system to a state of optimum balance and harmony.**

Alternative therapists are also likely to discuss additional issues, such as evaluating the quality of the diet and suggesting immune-boosting nutrients and supplements that could be added to it, or investigating stress-reduction techniques. This latter is particularly important since, as we have already seen, susceptibility to persistent infection can often follow a period of severe or excessively long-drawn-out emotional stress.

Some problems can be dealt with by the self-measures found in the following chapters, but there are specific indications that would suggest treatment from a trained therapist is more likely to yield successful results. If more than one of the following problems applies to you, there is a good chance that you would benefit greatly from a course of traditional Chinese medicine, Western medical herbalism, naturopathy, homeopathy or nutritional therapy.

- A general sense of mental and physical exhaustion with extremely poor energy levels that make it difficult to accomplish straightforward tasks at work and at home.
- More than one or two minor colds a year.
- Persistent skin rashes that appear periodically without ever clearing up completely.
- Periodical or persistent inflammation, pain, and swelling in the small joints of the fingers and toes.
- Swollen glands in the neck, armpits, and/or groin.
- Recurrent cold sores after a cold or when you are feeling run down.
- Generally poor skin tone and skin quality with a tendency to break out regularly in severe spots or boils.
- Recurrent problems with cystitis and/or thrush.

Problems with more than one of the above on a regular basis would suggest that your condition is "chronic". Many people mistakenly think that "chronic" refers to its severity when in fact, it is related more specifically to the recurring nature of the condition. For instance, if you are subject to persistent episodes of symptoms that refuse to clear up, no matter how much time and optimum support is given them, this would suggest a chronic problem. Excellent examples of chronic problems include migraines, thrush, irritable bowel syndrome, and asthma.

However, if a problem has severe symptoms that occur as an isolated incident and clear up of their own accord without any hint of returning, it falls into a category called "acute". Good examples of an acute illness include a one-off tension headache, hangover, episode of food poisoning, bout of 'flu or bruising following a fall.

A single episode of an acute problem should respond well to the measures outlined in the following chapters. This is because of the way that using alternative medicines for self-help purposes will speed up the process that would occur as a natural rule. The favourable result is that symptoms are reduced in duration and severity and are far less likely to leave complications behind them.

Most significantly of all, alternative medicines aim to restore the whole system to health, rather than attempting to eliminate specific micro-organisms with the risk of the attendant side effects outlined above. As a result, when alternative medical approaches are successful they should act gently, effectively and without the risk of serious side effects.

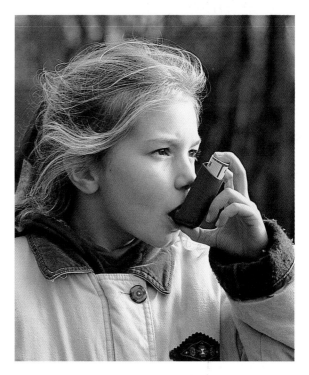

ABOVE: **Alternative treatments for chronic conditions such as asthma should always be provided by a trained practitioner.**

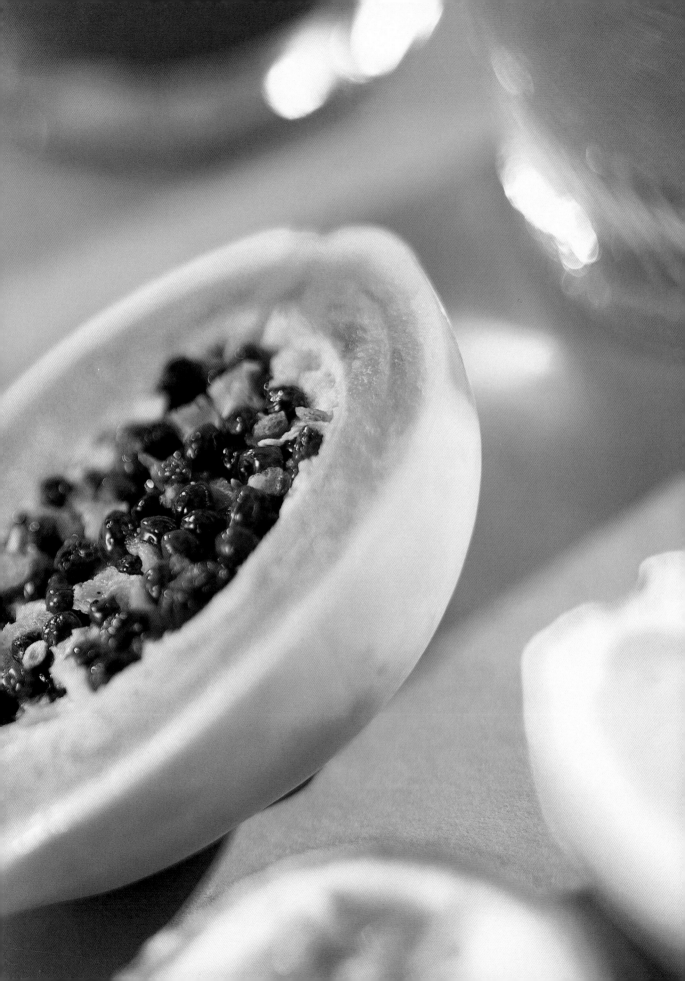

Many of us may feel that we are spoilt for choice when we consider how eating and food-shopping patterns have changed over the past twenty to thirty years. The variety of fast foods, international dishes and exotic ingredients available on the shelves of the average supermarket can seem quite overwhelming at times.

Our basic fascination with food is also reflected in the many television programmes devoted to virtually every aspect of cooking, from learning about the most basic techniques – such as how to boil the perfect egg! – to preparing Thai, Italian, French or Indian meals from scratch.

But wide availability and increased variety does not necessarily translate into a better diet. Because we have such an enticing variety of foods to choose from, we might be forgiven for assuming that we have never eaten as healthily as we do now. Sadly, this is not as true as it might initially seem as many common health problems that we suffer from can be linked to problems with our overall diet.

The trouble stems not so much from the variety of raw ingredients available to us as from what manufacturers do to those foods when processing them. Fast foods, snacks such as crisps and roasted salted nuts, fizzy drinks, tea, coffee, alcohol, chocolate, foods made from refined (white) sugar and flour, heavily preserved foods and foods with a high proportion of animal and hydrogenated fats will all contribute to a general level of lacklustre health when eaten on a regular basis.

The good news is that the reverse is also true and it is easy to put together an eating plan that will boost the immune system and enhance our general experience of health, vitality and well-being. The trick lies in knowing which foods are immune-system friendly and which are the opposite. Once we have got this clear in our minds, we are free to explore a vitality-enhancing diet that is delicious to eat and flexible enough to accommodate a healthy social life, as well as being packed with essential immunity-boosting nutrients.

The Basic Principles

The basic thinking behind devising an eating plan that gives the immune system a boost has a great deal in common with current general advice on healthy eating. Some of the small details may vary a little, but the most important points to remember are virtually the same. They are:

- Always choose foods that are as close to their natural state as possible, such as wholewheat products and brown rice and as many fresh, raw fruit and vegetables as possible. This is important because refining and preserving processes remove much of a food's nutritional potential. For example, by choosing to eat wholemeal bread we will be giving the body the chance to benefit

3
Boosting Immunity
through Nutrition

from the vitamins B and E and the healthy amounts of dietary fibre in the whole wheat grain. Products made from refined, white flour will be devoid of many nutritional benefits and also lack essential dietary fibre because the husk and wheatgerm of the whole grain are removed during processing. The same is true of many other grains, including rice: choosing brown over polished, white rice is always going to give us greater returns in the nutritional stakes.

- Avoid any foods that have been tampered with in order to extend their shelf-life. This includes any food that has been freeze-dried, vacuum-packed, canned, dehydrated or irradiated. Not only are foods that are prepared in this way often shockingly devoid of nutritional value, but most are also heavily laden with chemical additives, preservatives and colourings in order to improve their appearance and flavour – or at least to give a rough approximation of how the food looked and tasted when it was in its fresh state. The chemicals involved in these processes put a heavy burden on the body's organs of de-toxification and have a strongly compromising effect on the functioning of the immune system. Some of us may already be aware of this link if we have noticed that chemicals such as monosodium glutamate set off allergic symptoms such as digestive problems, headaches or sneezing with excessive production of mucus and

BELOW: **Aim for a minimum of five portions of fresh fruit and vegetables each day for maximum benefit to the immune system.**

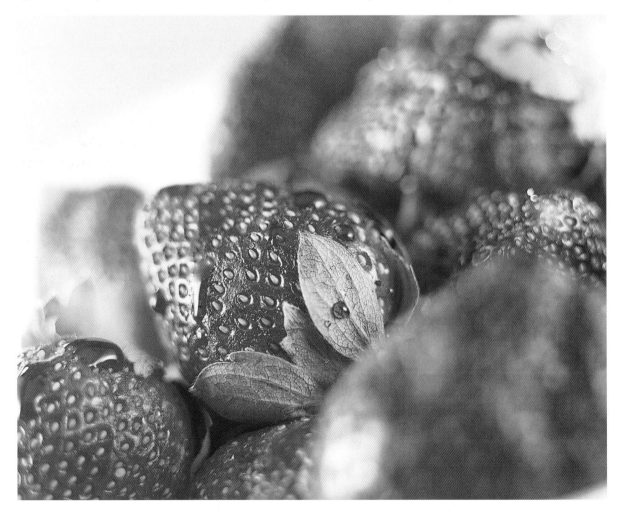

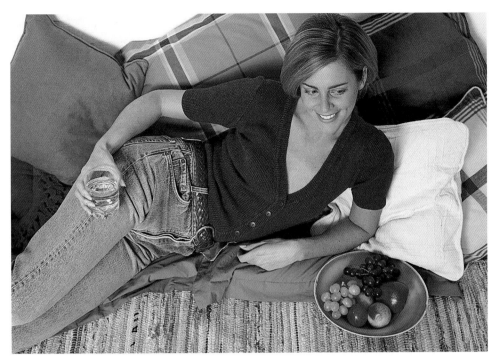

RIGHT: **Drinking regular amounts of still mineral water or spring water each day helps ensure that problems will not arise as a result of low-grade dehydration.**

catarrh. These are sure signs from our bodies that all is not well.

- Eat fresh vegetables and fruit frequently – they are packed with agents that will boost the immune system. To get maximum benefit from these fruits and vegetables they should be eaten every day. Remember that if it is difficult for any reason to eat at least five portions of fresh fruit and vegetables every day, juices (ideally freshly-squeezed) also count.

- Make sure that low-grade dehydration does not become a problem by drinking six large glasses of filtered tap water or still mineral water each day. Above all, don't make the mistake of thinking that tea, coffee or fizzy colas count as re-hydrating liquids. Apart from the additional health problems these drinks may cause, they act as diuretics, stimulating the body into getting rid of more liquid. As a result, they can contribute to problems with dehydration, rather than serving as an ally in combating this basic problem. If you suffer from an on-going problem with low-level dehydration you are likely to suffer from recurrent headaches, poor quality skin,

digestive problems and persistent constipation. When the last-named becomes a chronic problem, additional strain is placed on the body's organs of detoxification, which can have a subtle and persistent undermining effect on general health and on energy levels.

- Explore other forms of protein besides animal sources like red meat and dairy products. Although these are concentrated forms of complete protein, they can also bring a host of health problems with them when they are eaten in large quantities on a frequent basis. Experiment instead with small quantities of organic dairy produce and oily fish, eat frequent helpings of whole grains (such as brown rice) and beans and pulses. Combining these two food groupings gives the body the necessary complete form of protein it requires along with beneficial dietary fibre.

- Avoid foods and drinks containing refined (white) sugar as much as possible. However much of a challenge this might seem at first, it really is well worth the effort if we want to enjoy high-level immunity and vitality. Eating and drinking regular amounts of sugar in the form of

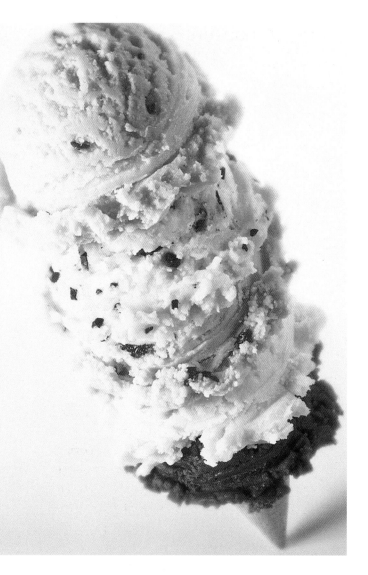

ABOVE: **Most commercially-prepared ice creams are alarmingly high in refined sugar and saturated fats.**

sugary foods eaten. Too much white sugar can also contribute to mood swings, stomach acidity and a tendency to suffer from recurrent thrush.

- Avoiding over-eating, especially if we avoid immune system-suppressing foods such as sugar, unhealthy fats from dairy sources or those that include immune system-suppressing trans-fatty acids, and red meat, does the immune system a huge favour. Concentrating instead on healthy portions of salads, fresh fruit, vegetables, pulses, grains, wholemeal products and oily fish, not only does the immune system a favour, but also helps avoid additional health problems such as heart disease that are associated with carrying extra, unwanted weight.

- Avoiding smoking is a must if we want to protect and support our immune systems. Cigarettes are known to bring a depressingly wide range of health problems with them, including increased risk of lung cancer, heart disease, chronic lung diseases such as bronchitis and osteoporosis (reduced bone density). In addition, smoking contributes to the production of free radicals in the body. Free radicals are profoundly reactive molecules that can damage or destroy other molecules in the body. They are believed to be intimately linked to signs of premature ageing, and can also leave us extremely vulnerable to degenerative diseases such as atherosclerosis, dementia and cancer. Free radicals appear to be a significant factor in the process of "cross-linking" of proteins which contributes to such cosmetic aspects of premature ageing as sagging and wrinkling of the skin. These rampaging molecules also have the potential to have a destructive effect on cellular levels, adversely affecting DNA and RNA so that we are more vulnerable to pre-cancerous changes occurring. As free radical production can also be stimulated in response to contact with a host of environmental toxins such as solvents, pesticides and radiation, we would do very well to reduce the load by making sure we avoid cigarette smoke, both by giving up smoking ourselves and by avoiding passive smoking whenever possible.

fizzy drinks, cakes, biscuits, chocolate, ice cream and savoury convenience foods, such as baked beans, that have a surprising amount of "hidden" sugar added to them, does nothing to improve our health. A diet that is high in refined sugar substantially increases the risk of developing obesity, heart disease, diabetes and dental cavities. In addition, sugar has been shown to have a significantly suppressive effect on the immune system, an effect that gets stronger with the proportion of

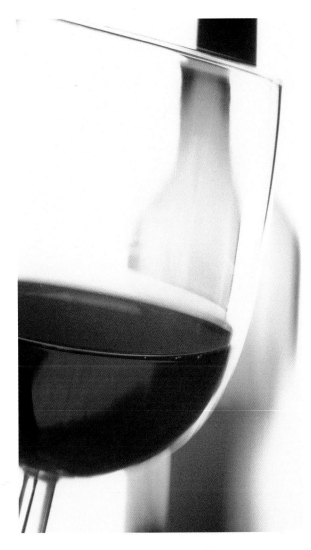

ABOVE: **A glass of red wine a day can be beneficial, but excessive amounts of alcohol can do serious damage to the liver.**

- Drink alcohol in moderation to avoid placing an undue amount of pressure on the body's primary organ of detoxification, the liver. Although a small amount of alcohol, such as a glass of red wine a day, can be beneficial to the circulatory system, drinking up to or in excess of recommended weekly alcohol allowances is sure to cause health problems. The maximum weekly allowance is fourteen units for women and twenty-one for men. One unit is a small glass of wine, a standard measure of spirits or a half a pint of beer or lager.

Immune-boosting Foods

Here are some of the basic ingredients that need to be added to your daily diet if you want to boost and protect the performance of your immune system. Do remember that what is being aimed for here is a basic framework that can be adopted on a long-term basis in order to experience optimum health and vitality. The suggestions made are deliberately not extreme or drastic, but should be easy to stick to without feeling restricted or hard-pressed to know what to eat.

Most significantly of all, the emphasis is on outlining what can be added to the diets rather offering a harsh list of what has to be eliminated. It is also flexible, so that if you temporarily go slightly off course – on holiday or during the Christmas party season, for instance – you will know how to get back on track as quickly and effectively as possible.

Always remember that to gain the maximum benefit from what you eat, you should never lose sight of the sensual pleasure that food gives. This has to be a central part of any eating plan that is going to work on a long-term basis. Of course, the basic principles can be applied in a more drastic way if you want to kick off with a more radical start by de-toxing your system. But in the main, it helps to remember that drastic measures that are not followed by a long-term change in eating patterns are only likely to give short-term returns. A more realistic, achievable approach will give the basic framework needed to make your eating patterns a health bonus rather than a health hazard.

Remember, too, that the way foods are prepared can be almost as important as the quality of the ingredients themselves when it comes to making the most of their immunity-boosting potential.

Fresh Fruit and Green Vegetables

In any immunity-boosting eating plan, it is essential to have as many helpings of fresh, raw fruit and vegetables as you can manage. Although the choice available varies slightly according to the season, there is still an impressively wide range of fruit and vegetables available to us most of the time in large supermarkets. There is such a wide variety of choice on offer that fruit and vegetables can easily be chosen to suit your mood, budget, and time available on any given day. They can be included in salads, soups, purées, freshly-blended pasta sauces, home-made fruit and vegetable juices, casseroles, couscous and bite-sized snacks made from sticks of chopped raw fruit and vegetables.

The benefits to the immune system of including frequent helpings of fruit and vegetables are multiple, and are partly connected to the antioxidant nutrients in dark orange, yellow, red and green vegetables. More information about antioxidants is given in the following chapter and all you need to know at this stage is that they help us fight the negative effects of free radicals in our bodies. As a result, they appear to play an important role in protecting us against a host of degenerative diseases, as well as having anti-ageing properties.

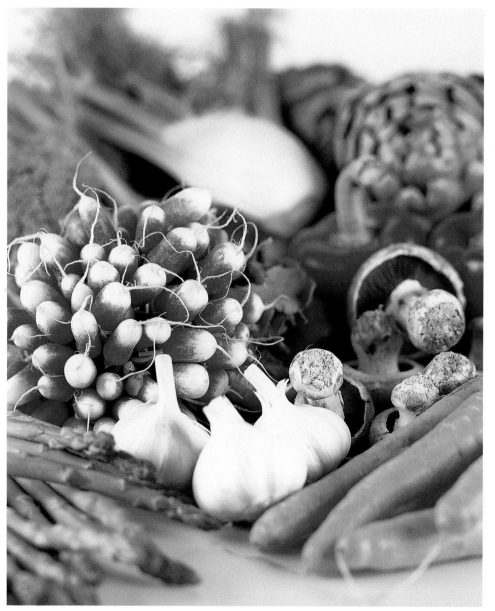

LEFT: **Orange, red and green vegetables are rich sources of antioxidant nutrients which play an essential role in boosting the good functioning of the immune system.**

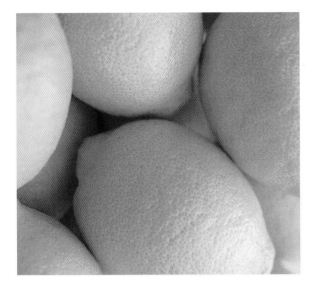

ABOVE: **Lemons, like other citrus fruits, are excellent sources of vitamin C, a nutrient essential for good health and the proper functioning of the immune system.**

CITRUS FRUITS

It is well known that citrus fruits such as oranges, lemons and grapefruit contain lots of vitamin C. Less well-known, perhaps, is the fact that there are alternative sources of this essential nutrient and supporter of the immune system available in other fruit and vegetables, including kiwifruit, dark red or purple berries such as blueberries, tomatoes, peppers and dark green vegetables. This is especially good news for those who may have food sensitivities that include negative reactions to citrus fruits.

FRUITS CONTAINING LYCOPENE

Tomatoes, watermelons, guavas and grapefruit are rich in the carotenoid lycopene. This is a fat-soluble nutrient which appears to have a powerful action on the immune system which may protect against cancer. Because of olive oil's fat-soluble nature, adding a little cold-pressed olive oil to tomatoes before eating them appears to allow the body a greater uptake of the lycopene in the tomatoes.

GRAPES

Grapes appear to have an important role to play in protecting against cancer because of the presence of an important phytochemical called reservatrol. They are also sources of selenium and quercetin. Possible benefits of eating grapes frequently include lowered cholesterol levels, reduced incidence of allergies and improved condition of the circulatory system. For maximum benefits, choose red or purple grapes in preference to green as they appear to have a higher antioxidant yield.

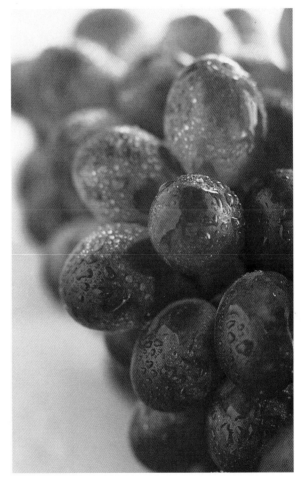

ABOVE: **Red and purple grape varieties yield good levels of important antioxidants with valuable health benefits.**

CRUCIFEROUS VEGETABLES

Cruciferous vegetables such as broccoli, cauliflower, cabbage, and watercress are generating interest among nutritionists because of the protection they appear to give against cancer of the colon and breast and intestinal polyps. The

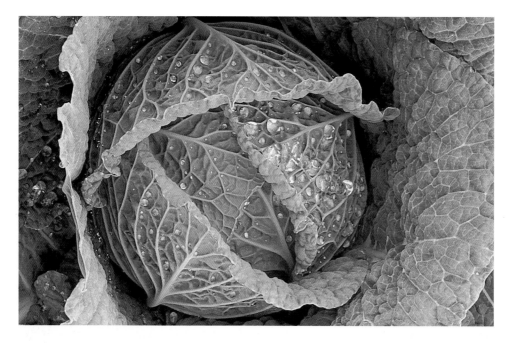

LEFT: **Dark green vegetables, such as cabbages, appear to give extra protection against cancer and also boost dietary fibre intake.**

phytochemicals found in broccoli appear to have a positive effect in switching off cancer cells and allowing the body to eliminate them. The sulphoraphane that broccoli also contains appears to support helper T-cells in identifying cancer cells so that they can be dealt with as speedily as possible.

DIETARY FIBRE

Fruit and vegetables are an essential source of dietary fibre, which plays an important role in protecting against chronic digestive problems such as constipation. A diet that is seriously low in fibre can leave us more vulnerable to obesity and to diseases of the heart and bowel. It is thought that the high-fibre content of a healthy vegetarian diet may be one of the important factors in vegetarians having a substantially reduced risk of dying of cancer. It has been estimated that this may be approximately 40 per cent lower than for meat eaters.

Healthy Fats

Many people have been persuaded that if something is said to be a "low-fat" product it must be healthy. This is very far from the truth. Commercially produced low-fat foods are far too often packed with chemical additives that do very little to enhance health, and may, indeed, play a significant role in undermining it. This has a particular relevance when we talk about boosting the immune system as immunity-friendly foods – whole grains, fruit, vegetables and fresh, unroasted nuts and seeds – tend to be as close to their natural state as possible .

Look at the list of ingredients on an average low-fat, reduced-sugar, or reduced-calorie product and you are likely to be amazed at the number of chemical additives such as preservatives, flavourings and colourings that are used in it. If you are concerned about reducing your contact with immunity-depressing or potentially toxic chemicals, you would do well to avoid any foods that have been tampered with to this extent.

As for the fats themselves, it is true that protecting the body from conditions such as high blood pressure, heart disease and breast cancer involves strictly limiting intakes of saturated fats that are found in such foods as butter, cream, cheese and red meat. However, the body needs a balanced intake of essential fats to remain in good health.

ESSENTIAL FATTY ACIDS

Healthy fats and oils that are rich in essential fatty acids (EFAs) are necessary for protection against heart disease and to help guard against hormone imbalance as well as lowering the risk of developing cancer. These "friendly" fats, needed for optimum health, are to be found in seeds, nuts, and cold-pressed, unrefined, virgin oils. Oily fish, olives, whole grains and dark green vegetables are also rich sources of EFAs.

When EFAs and the sterols and sterolins found in flaxseed oil and olive oil are combined with a diet containing plenty of fresh vegetables and fruits, the immune system is being given exactly the support it needs to work at optimum efficiency, fighting infection, controlling candida proliferation and keeping tumours at bay. If the body has a regular supply of EFAs, hormone-type substances called prostaglandins are helped to guard against inflammatory conditions flaring up, and will prevent obvious or severe symptoms of pre-menstrual syndrome.

However, this is all a matter of balance as if too many foods that contain unhealthy, saturated fats are eaten, prostaglandins will leave the body vulnerable to developing inflammatory conditions and pre-menstrual symptoms.

USING VEGETABLE OILS

When choosing vegetable oils, opt for cold-pressed, virgin varieties of olive, sunflower or safflower oils sold in glass containers. Avoid buying any vegetable oils in plastic containers, since residues of chemicals from the plastic can leach into the oil. Once opened, oils should be stored in dark-coloured glass bottles out of direct sunlight in order to prevent them becoming oxidized or damaged. Always reject refined, odourless and tasteless oils that have been processed to such a degree that vital immunity-boosting phytonutrients will have been removed just to give the oil a more cosmetically-appealing clarity.

Be especially wary of heating solid fats made from vegetable oils to a high temperature for cooking, since this can contribute to free radical production. Also avoid heating commercially prepared oils to very high temperatures since this damages the EFAs in polyunsaturated oils.

There are additional problems associated with hydrogenated vegetable fats that are solid at room temperature. This is because the process of hydrogenating vegetable oils to

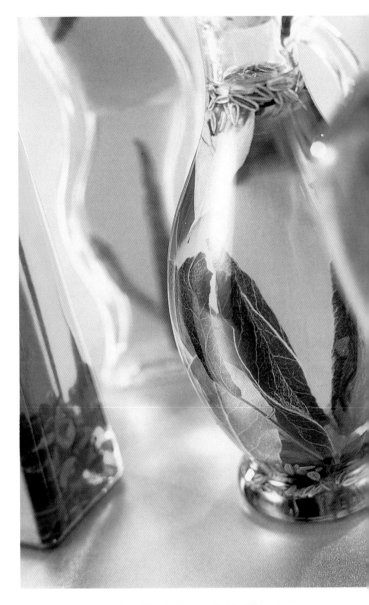

ABOVE: **Keep a few good-quality oils flavoured with different herbs and spices in the kitchen to add extra interest to cooking.**

make them solid – heating them to high temperatures and passing hydrogen through them – causes the formation of dangerous trans-fatty acids. These trans-fatty acids bear a resemblance to the saturated fats in foods like butter, cheese and red meat. As a result, they may cause health hazards similar to those caused by saturated fats when they are used regularly and in generous quantities.

CHOOSING THE BEST FATS

There are several ways of ensuring that your diet contains a healthy balance of fats:

- Eat very sparing quantities of butter in preference to generous quantities of margarine. Avoid low-fat spreads made from unhealthy trans-fatty acids.
- Boost healthy EFA intake by including oily fish, such as fresh salmon and mackerel, walnuts and pumpkin seeds in the diet.
- Cut down fairly drastically on saturated fats. This can be done very effectively by strictly reducing the amount of red meat, full-fat cheese, full-fat milk and cream that you eat.
- Always choose virgin, cold-pressed olive or sunflower oils, which contain healthy EFAs that protect the heart and circulatory system, for cooking. Use these beneficial, unsaturated oils in salad dressings, combining them with a little lemon juice or vinegar.

Green Tea and Other Herb Teas

Green tea (drunk without milk) is attracting an increasing amount of attention as a healthy alternative to caffeinated drinks such as coffee, black tea, hot chocolate and colas. Caffeinated drinks can bring a host of problems with them when drunk on a regular basis, including sleep disturbance, jitteriness, breast tenderness, recurrent headaches, persistent fatigue and elevated blood pressure. Anyone at high risk of developing osteoporosis (reduced bone density) should also treat caffeinated drinks with caution because regular intakes of caffeine can result in magnesium deficiency as the caffeine stimulates the mineral's excretion from the body.

Substituting green tea – ideally organic – for caffeinated beverages such as coffee gives the body regular exposure to immunity-boosting antioxidants and bioflavonoids, which appear to play a significant role in helping the body fight bacterial and viral infections.

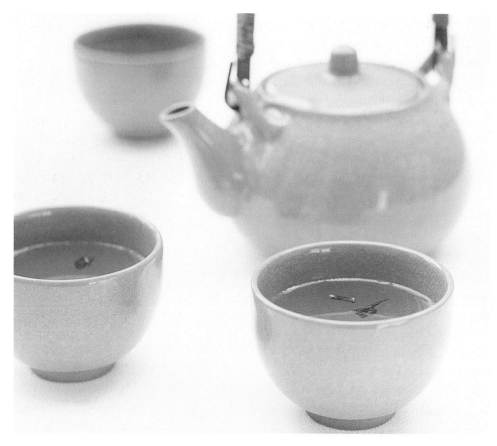

RIGHT: **Green tea is free of the caffeine of standard black tea. It can be bought in many of the popular flavour blends of ordinary tea.**

A good way to ring the changes with hot beverages is to explore the wide range of fruit and herbal teas available, experimenting with different ones until you discover ones you really enjoy. You may respond best to the soothing qualities of camomile or peppermint tea or instinctively prefer the zingy, stimulating citrus fruit teas available.

Garlic

Garlic appears to have an amazingly wide beneficial effect on the immune system, including providing potential benefits in fighting bacterial, fungal and viral infections, reducing inflammation, and benefiting the heart and the circulatory system. Research suggests that the protective and health-promoting effects of garlic may be linked to its allicin content, although garlic also contains a wide range of compounds which appear to have a part to play in the well-being of the mind and the body.

The sulfur compounds in garlic are considered to be the main source of its immune system-boosting effect, because of the way in which they support the action of killer cells. Taking garlic regularly is thought to enhance the immune system's potential for eliminating cancer cells and bacterial and viral infections. Garlic is also a must for those who are prone to recurring infections that seem to need regular courses of antibiotics to overcome as garlic appears to offer a genuine, effective alternative antibacterial treatment.

If you enjoy the flavour of garlic, add it to roasted vegetables, casseroles and stews, or bake it on its own in a garlic baker to provide a delicious and original side vegetable dish. For those who have reservations about its pungent taste and smell or who find that it disagrees with them, there are several alternative ways of enjoying the health-promoting benefits of garlic (see page 68).

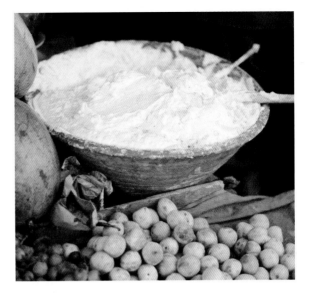

ABOVE: **Live, natural yoghurt is a rich source of probiotics that help keep the digestive system in balance.**

Yoghurt

Probiotics have been attracting a great deal of attention recently as being essential allies in our efforts to enhance immunity. The immune system can be both weakened and suppressed by over-use of antibiotics, especially when taken within the context of an overall poor nutritional status. With the immune system constantly needing to defend itself against viruses and antibiotic-resistant strains of increasingly powerful bacteria, it clearly needs all the help it can get in supporting the body's defensive battles effectively.

One of the ways to provide this support is through supplementing the daily diet with the probiotics that can be found in live, natural yoghurt. Yoghurts containing acidophilus appear to inhibit the reproduction of viruses, while also having the beneficial effect of reducing inflammation in the gut. When lactobacillus bulgaricus is taken on a regular basis, it has powerful antibacterial properties while also enhancing the parasite-eliminating effect of the immunoglobulin IgE.

The probiotics found in live yoghurt have a beneficial effect on the gut by helping to balance the friendly micro-organisms needed for the smooth working of the digestive tract. Digestive disturbances such as diarrhoea that commonly occur after a course of antibiotics may be eased by taking probiotic-enriched yoghurt.

Adding a cup of probiotic-enriched yoghurt to your daily diet appears to be a simple and painless way of ensuring that you are supporting your body's defences.

Shiitake and Reishi Mushrooms

Shiitake mushrooms, sold fresh by most supermarkets, are rich in a broad spectrum of phytochemicals, including the amino acids leucine, lysine and threonine, as well as calcium, phosphorus and vitamin D. In addition, they appear to have a powerful immune system-booster in the form of lentinan. This appears to stimulate the production of interferon, which helps the body fight viral infections more effectively. It also appears to have an impact in helping keep tumours at bay, thus possibly reducing the risk of cancer.

Reishi mushrooms (available in capsule or tincture form) appear to have a broad spectrum of positive action, and are used in Chinese medicine to treat patients suffering from hepatitis, bronchitis, bronchial asthma, gastric ulcers, migraine and coronary

ABOVE: **Shiitake mushrooms contain valuable phytochemicals and also lentinan, a booster for the immune system.**

heart disease. Reishi mushrooms have been shown to have adaptogenic properties that have a positive impact on regulating blood sugar levels, boosting immune-system functioning, combating free radical activity, regulating blood pressure and lowering cholesterol. They also have a natural sedative effect.

Because of the tough and largely indigestible nature of reishi mushrooms, they need to be cooked and processed before the potential of their medicinal qualities can be released. This is why, unlike shiitake mushrooms, they are best take in medicinal form.

Eating for Maximum Immunity: A Quick Tour

This section outlines an approach to eating that gives long-term benefit and support to the immune system. It is a three-way approach, emphasizing the best kinds of food to eat, and also indicating those foods which are best included in the plan occasionally or avoided as much as possible.

When the "best" foods form the staple part of a daily diet, they give the body the best chance of performing as smoothly and effectively as possible. The beauty of this approach to nutrition is its flexibility: it allows for plans to go slightly off course. There is no need to feel so completely demoralized that you give up because you can't keep to a strict and rigid plan. All you have to do is get back on track within the general boundaries given below.

Essential Foods

These are the types of food that are essential in any plan for eating for maximum immunity.

- Fish of all kinds, but especially oily fish that are high in EFAs. These should be cooked in low-fat ways such as baking, steaming or stir-frying in a small amounts of cold-pressed, virgin olive oil. Avoid battered or deep-fried fish whenever possible.
- Fresh soups, ideally homemade, using any vegetables in

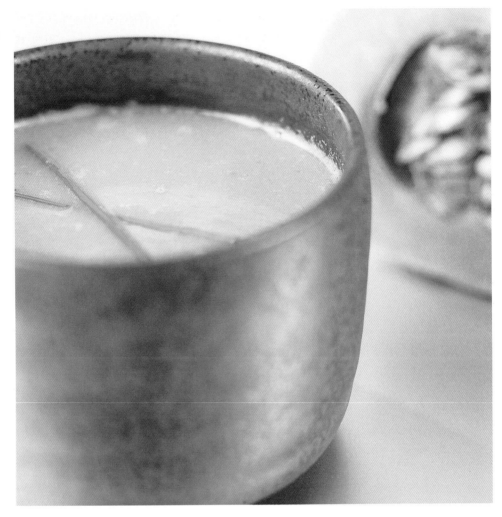

RIGHT: **Freshly made soups, such as this rich pumpkin soup, are a delicious way of boosting your in take of fresh vegetables and pulses.**

season. Add whole grains and pulses in winter for extra bulk, texture and flavour.

- Fresh fruit and vegetables – at least five servings a day. Choose from as wide a variety as possible. Fruit and vegetables can be eaten in many ways – raw as salads, lightly cooked as side dishes, as crudités for crunchy snacks, as fresh fruit juices or puréed as accompaniments to main dishes – so you will never be bored by them.
- Wholewheat pasta and brown rice.
- Pulses and beans. Try using them in Indian dishes which are especially delicious and spicy, guaranteed to give the lie to the still prevalent idea that vegetarian food must be worthy and bland.

- Sauces based on concentrated tomato, which is very rich in lycopene, are excellent with brown rice, pasta and baked potatoes. Add other vegetables and fresh herbs according to taste.
- Salad dressings, made from cold-pressed olive or sunflower oils with vinegar or lemon juice, or natural bio yoghurt blended with herbs.
- White meat such as chicken or turkey. Always choose organic poultry where possible, since the term "free range" is not a guarantee that the birds will not have had drugs or other chemicals added to their food. "Free range" applies to the surroundings in which the birds are kept rather than to the way in which they are fed.

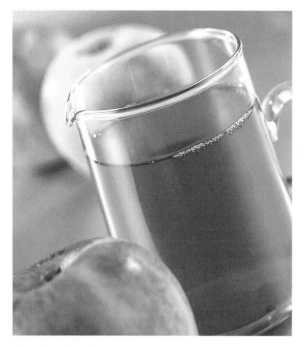

ABOVE: **Freshly-squeezed fruit juices count as part of your daily fruit intake. Fruit put through a juicer retains much of its fibre.**

- Natural bio yoghurt. This is delicious on its own, but variety can be introduced by adding natural spices such as cinnamon or chopped fresh fruit.
- Fresh fruit juices or blended "smoothies". Use fresh fruit in season, adding natural bio yoghurt for added texture and bulk. Make fresh vegetable juices, too: vegetables are especially rich in antioxidants.
- Regular amounts of still mineral or filtered tap water drunk through the day. Aim to drink at least five to six glasses every day, taking a bottle to work in order to keep a check on how much has been drunk during the day.
- Green tea.
- Garlic. Add it regularly in a generous way to sauces and vegetable dishes and grate it raw into salad dressings.
- Semi-skimmed organic milk.
- Sparing amounts of organic butter in preference to hydrogenated vegetable spreads.
- Rice cakes made from organic brown rice. These can be bought glazed with soy sauce and garlic or with savoury, yeast-based flavourings.

Occasional Foods

Include these foods occasionally in your immunity-boosting eating plan.

- Cheeses such as Edam, Jarlsberg, Camembert, Gouda, fromage frais and some ewe's or goat's cheese.
- Organic, free-range eggs. Eat these boiled, scrambled or poached but never fried.
- Alcohol, drunk within moderate limits, and choosing a glass of red or dry white wine in preference to spirits, beer or lager.
- Organic cakes and biscuits.
- Chocolate as an occasional treat, always choosing organic.
- Red meat. If you find it very hard to give up red meat altogether, choose organically farmed produce. Make a point of avoiding eating red meat on consecutive nights,

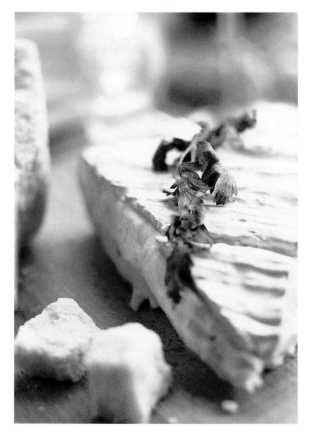

ABOVE: **Cheese should always be eaten sparingly, because of its high saturated fat content.**

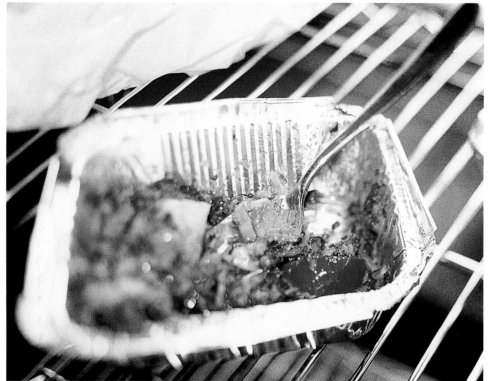

choosing instead to make fish, white meat, and regular portions of pulses and whole grains the mainstay of your diet. By restricting yourself to occasional helpings of red meat on an infrequent basis, there is less chance of a toxic build-up occurring, caused by the way that red meat travels slowly through the digestive tract, with the result that it can putrefy before it has a chance to be eliminated from the body.

- Coffee or tea. Avoid decaffeinated coffee that uses chemical solvents to remove the caffeine content, since these chemicals can be toxic. When using decaffeinated coffee choose brands that are known to use a water filtering process instead. Alternatively, opt for drinks that contain guarana, green tea, or herbal and fruit teas.
- Reduced-fat crème fraîche.

Foods to Avoid

Some kinds of food should be avoided as much as possible.

- Any processed foods that are dehydrated, preserved with chemicals, canned or vacuum-packed: in other words, most "instant" snacks or meals that suggest all you have to do is add water and stir.
- Items that are very high in fat, such as pâté, sausages, smoked meat or salami. Apart from their generous fat content, such foods also tend to be high in salt and additives such as phosphorous (often listed on food labels as sodium phosphate, potassium phosphate, or phosphoric acid). These are best avoided if you want to look after your immune system to the best of your ability.
- Convenience foods made from refined (white) flour and sugar, especially if they also contain a generous portion of saturated or hydrogenated fat. Manufactured foods that tend to contain all three of these ingredients include cakes, biscuits and puddings.
- Foods that have been irradiated or based on ingredients that have been genetically modified.
- Indian or Chinese take-away meals. These really should be a very infrequent treat rather than a regular feature of

the diet. Indian take-away dishes tend to contain large amounts of saturated fats and Chinese dishes use chemical flavourings and colourings. If Indian and Chinese foods are favourites, make your own. Enjoy healthy homemade Chinese stir-fries, quickly made using a little cold-pressed olive oil and chopped vegetables, seafood, poultry, or fish. Delicious Indian dishes can also be made at home using bio yoghurt, pulses, and fresh vegetables.

- "Diet" drinks and foods that have had artificial sweeteners such as saccharine or aspartame added. Apart from tasting unpleasant, these artificial sweeteners are known to be a health hazard, and are best avoided whenever possible.
- Saturated fat in the form of cream or soured cream.
- Potato crisps and roasted salted peanuts, and cashews (especially when they have a hefty amount of sugar added in a honey glaze as well as salt).

Getting Down to Practicalities

Knowing what foods you should be eating is just a first step. It is also important to know about choosing, preparing and cooking the ingredients.

Choosing and Preparing Food

You need to pay attention to the quality of the food you buy if you are to get maximum nutritional support from it. These basic points will help you select the best possible fresh fruit and vegetables:

- Choose organic vegetables whenever possible, especially root vegetables and potatoes. This is particularly important since residues from chemicals can be absorbed as deep as 50mm (¼ inch) beneath the skin. Many nutrients in potatoes are stored just beneath the skin, which is why they are best cooked and eaten unpeeled. The problem is that boiling non-organic potatoes in their skins can drive toxic chemicals further into the flesh.
- Don't be put off by the less-than-perfect appearance of

RIGHT: **Don't always buy the "tried and tested": ring the changes – artichokes instead of beans – when choosing vegetables.**

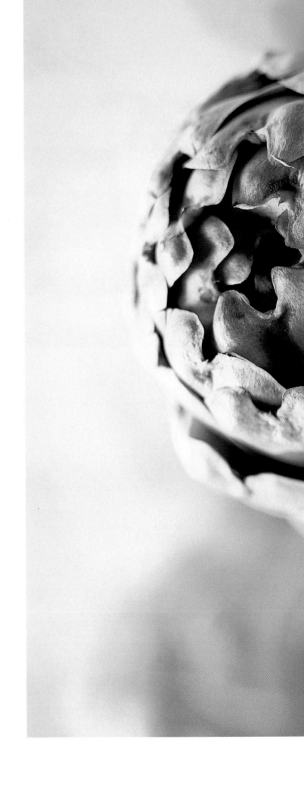

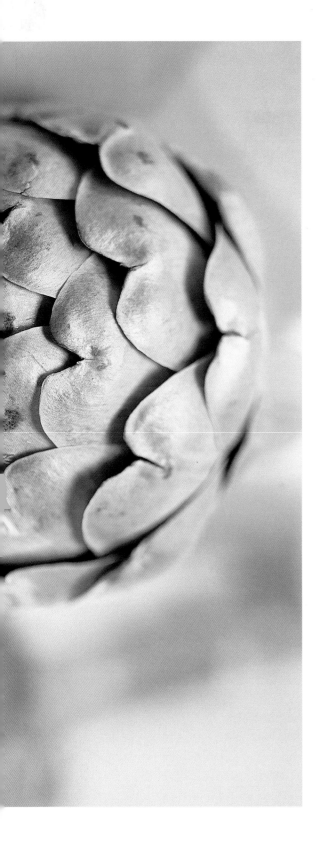

many organic fruits and vegetables. It is the price that we pay for the cultivation of produce without chemical pesticides and fertilizers. While the debate about the pros and cons of organic versus non-organic food continues, there is a persuasive argument that suggests that items grown without exposure to artificial chemical fertilizers and pesticides are likely to be of greater nutritional value.

- Avoid fruit and vegetables that look too perfect or appear and feel waxy to the touch. These can be tell-tale signs of chemical residues left on the skin.

- It is generally safer to peel or scrub non-organic vegetables thoroughly before cooking, to avoid any chemical residues being eaten with them.

- Eat as many raw portions of fresh fruit and vegetables as possible each day. Eating them uncooked preserves their vitamin C content, much of which is lost in cooking. Vitamin C oxidizes quickly when fruit and vegetables are chopped, so they should be prepared as close as possible to the time they are to be eaten. Always scrub or peel non-organic fruit and vegetables before eating them.

Cooking Food Healthily

In considering the issue of optimum nutrition, there is little point in discussing ingredients without paying attention to the way in which they are cooked. This is extremely important, because a very healthy ingredient can be turned into a health hazard if it is cooked in an unhealthy way.

For instance, if organic, scrubbed potatoes are baked in their skins they are an excellent source of complex carbohydrate. If the same potatoes are turned into french fries they become positively unhealthy. This is especially the case if refined vegetable oil is used for deep frying as it will have been heated to a very high temperature, thus increasing your exposure to free radicals. In addition, the amount of fat absorbed by fried potatoes is not beneficial to the heart or the circulatory system. Similar problems arise if potatoes are mashed with lashings of salt, butter and full-fat milk.

There is no need to feel discouraged, however, because there is a great range of cooking methods that preserve the nutritional value of food.

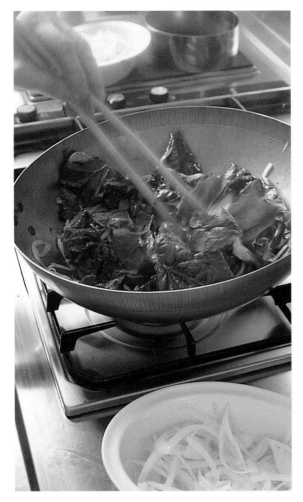

ABOVE: **Stir-frying preserves the texture, flavour and crispness of raw ingredients as well as their nutritional value.**

STIR-FRYING

This is a quick, versatile method of cooking that preserves the texture and nutritional value of foods and is a particularly attractive method for those for whom time is tight and who prefer to be spontaneous in their cooking, rather than slavishly following complicated recipe instructions. Stir-frying makes the most of ingredients such as shellfish, poultry, fish and a wide range of vegetables by stir-frying them in a small amount of cold-pressed, virgin olive oil and adding a flavouring such as a dash of soy sauce or fresh herbs. Because of the sparing amount of oil needed, stir-frying avoids the health hazards of deep frying, while also giving us the health-

protective benefits that come with using unsaturated oils such as unrefined olive or sunflower oils.

STEAMING

This is always the best way of lightly cooking vegetables in order to preserve their colour, texture and nutritional content. This is in sharp contrast to boiling, which encourages a significant proportion of vitamins to leach into the cooking water, though boiling is not quite such a loss if the cooking liquid is saved to make stocks or sauces. Steamers can be used to cook other ingredients, such as fish, that has a particularly delicate flavour or texture.

GRILLING

An excellent cooking method for meat or fish that needs to be done quickly or lightly. Use a rack or griddle that allows excess fat to drain away and avoid brushing any additional fat on to the food before cooking, unless absolutely necessary.

ROASTING

Like stir-frying and grilling, this is a healthy way of cooking meat, because no fat is needed other than the fat that is in the meat itself. High-fat meats such as lamb should be put on a rack so that fat from it can drip into the pan.

BROWNING OR SHALLOW FRYING

This is best done in a heavy pan over a steady, medium heat with no oil added, or with just a sparing amount of virgin, cold-pressed olive or sunflower oil for any items that don't exude their own juices during cooking.

Cooking Methods to Avoid

Some ways of cooking food can do appreciable damage to its nutritional value, and should be avoided.

DEEP-FRYING

This involves submerging food, sometimes covered with a hefty coating of a white-flour batter, in very hot cooking oil and should always be given the cold shoulder. This is especially the case with spongy vegetables such as mushrooms and

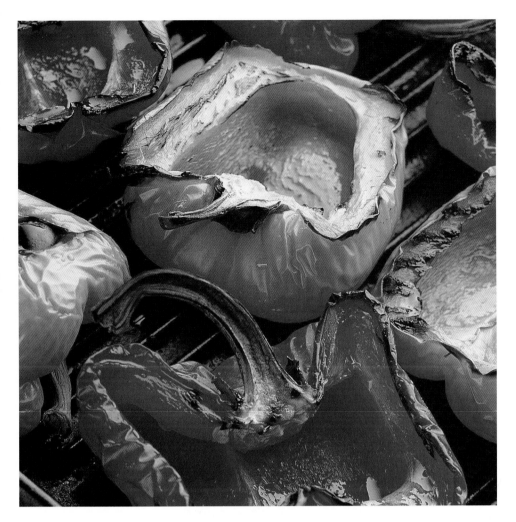

aubergines that quickly become saturated with cooking fat. We already know about the drawbacks associated with an unhealthy intake of dietary fat, so why add unnecessary amounts in this way?

BOILING

Cooking food in lots of water is always to be avoided if it needs to be served crisp and full of flavour. Tasteless, soggy heaps of cabbage, cauliflower or other vegetables are not just off-putting, they also lack many of their nutrients, lost into the cooking water. Only boil foods that cannot be cooked safely any other way, such as red kidney beans which must be thoroughly cooked, and at a high temperature for at least a part of the cooking time, before being eaten.

MICROWAVING

Cooking vegetables and other foods in a microwave oven is quick and convenient and preserves the colour, crisp texture and a significant proportion of the vitamin content. We should consider that however convenient microwaving might be as a cooking method, it would be wise not to rely too much on it as a basic cooking technique. We do not yet know what the long-term effects of eating microwaved foods might be on the body, nor do we know what the consequences might be of the molecular changes food goes through when it is microwaved.

There are also concerns over low-grade emissions from microwave ovens, so it would seem wise not to stand too close to a microwave oven while it is on, and to leave food to stand for a few seconds before opening the door once cooking is over.

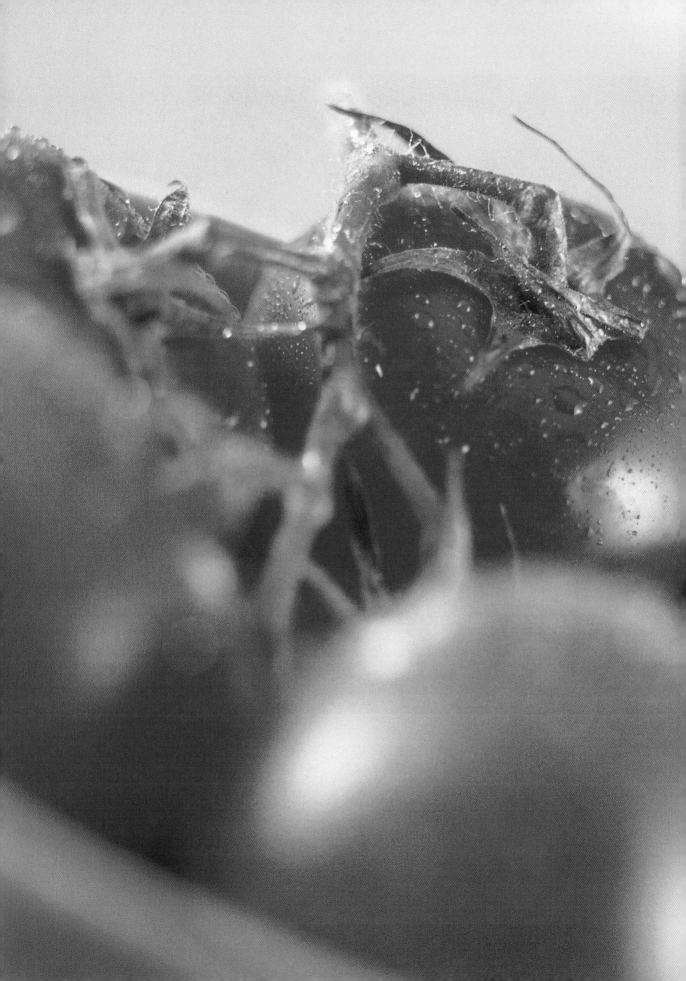

The debate about whether the average diet needs to be supplemented with vitamins and minerals is a heated one. Many nutritionists feel that people who are exposed to toxic chemicals, pollutants and low-grade radiation on a daily basis, whose diet is nutritionally poor because it is made up mainly of convenience foods, and who experience high levels of all-round stress, need extra back-up from taking regular, appropriate vitamin and mineral supplements.

An alternative view is that it is foolish to waste money on supplements that at best are not needed, and at worst may do some harm if toxic mega-doses become stored in the body. This view is based on the notion that an average "balanced" diet should yield all the basic nutrients we need.

As is so often the case with complex and emotive issues, the reality of the issue would seem to rest somewhere between these two opposing views. For people who live a hectic life with very little time to spare, who don't feel able to eat as healthily as they would like, and who suffer recurrent minor infections, taking appropriate nutritional supplements would seem to be an appropriate course of action.

On the other hand, those of us who eat at least five portions of organic fruit and vegetables a day, make a point of eating nutritionally sound food on a regular basis, have enough time to relax and exercise regularly, fight off minor infections vigorously and well and feel generally very positive about our lives, may get by very well without help from additional nutritional supplements.

It is likely, however, that even those of us who generally keep our lives running along healthy, balanced lines will find that there are times when we experience pressures and changes of routine that suggest we need extra help from appropriate nutritional supplements. These experiences could include any of the following:

- A period of acute emotional stress or shock such as coping with bereavement, unexpected redundancy or the break-up of a relationship.
- Physical stress and unusual emotional pressure resulting from working unusually long hours for an extended period of time.
- Pregnancy and giving birth.
- The menopause.
- A protracted or severe viral illness.

In any of these situations, following a programme of appropriate nutritional supplements can provide the essential boost needed to get us back on fighting form again.

Antioxidants and the Immune System

There is a specific group of nutrients that need to be considered before any other by anyone concerned about boosting the immune system when it appears to be flagging.

Boosting Immunity
with Antioxidants,
Vitamins & Minerals

4

Collectively, these nutrients are called antioxidants, and include the vitamins A, C and E and the mineral selenium. Antioxidants have been hailed as "super nutrients" that have the potential powerfully to protect the body against a wide range of degenerative illnesses, such as angina, stroke, lung cancer, coronary heart disease and dementia.

Antioxidants also appear to play an important role in preventing the body develop problems associated with premature ageing, and help fight minor infections on a day-to-day basis by giving the immune system valuable extra support.

Free radicals have already been considered for the negative role they can play in undermining overall health (see page 38). We now need to take a closer and more detailed look at the significance of an excess of free radicals in the body, since they are of central importance in any discussion of the relevance of antioxidants to the smooth and healthy functioning of the immune system.

THE THREAT OF FREE RADICALS

Free radicals are rampaging molecules that interfere with normal cellular activity in the body. When free-radical activity goes unchecked it can result in potentially severe damage to and deterioration of body tissues. Some free-radical activity within the body is a basic fact of life, because these destructive molecules are produced whenever oxygen is converted into energy, in a process is called oxidation.

Although the body needs to produce a certain number of free radicals in order to kill off harmful bacteria, once they begin to be produced in excessive amounts they have the unfortunate effect of leaving the body vulnerable to the development of degenerative disease.

The destructive effect of free radicals is related to their highly volatile and unstable nature which causes them to have a disruptive effect on cell membranes. It also allows them to tamper negatively with genetic material, causing a negative chain reaction that can cause severe damage to body tissues. These cellular terrorists have been cited as predisposing us to a disturbing number of serious diseases, including various cancers, heart disease, circulatory disorders, auto-immune problems such as rheumatoid arthritis and chronic neurological diseases such as Parkinson's Disease.

As more is learned about free radicals and their destructive potential, certain lifestyle choices are being highlighted as likely to elevate the risk of excessive free radical production. These include:

- Drinking more than moderate amounts of alcohol.
- Relying on excessive amounts of convenience and heavily-processed foods.
- Eating deep-fried foods regularly.
- Smoking (either actively or passively).
- Excessive, unprotected exposure to radiation from the sun.
- Exposure to atmospheric pollution such as car exhaust fumes or toxic chemicals in the work place.

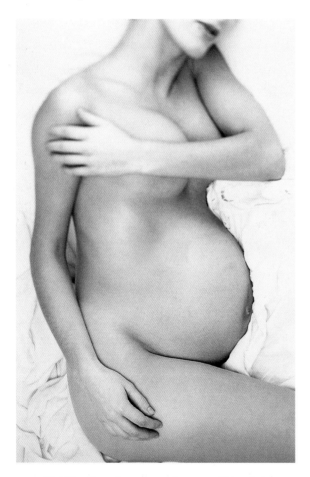

ABOVE: **Nutritional supplements may have a positive role to play in helping women who feel rundown following childbirth.**

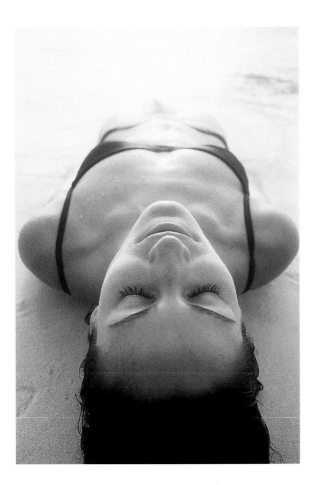

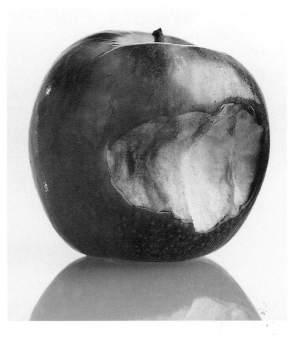

ABOVE: **The brown coating that has developed on this partly eaten apple is a sure sign that oxidation is at work.**

LEFT: **Too much unprotected sunbathing can have an adverse effect on health by causing premature ageing of the skin.**

When we are enjoying optimum health and our bodies are working in a balanced way due to a vigorous inherited constitution that is backed up by a health-promoting lifestyle, we should be able to keep free radicals in check by the body's in-built safety mechanisms.

On the other hand, if we are exposed to regular and excessive amounts of atmospheric pollution, coupled with severe and unrelieved stress levels, to which a poor diet and frequent exposure to cigarette smoke are added, there is a very good chance that we are going to end up with more free radicals circulating in our systems than we can effectively deal with. This is where antioxidant help can be invaluable in getting us back on track – provided, of course, we also generally cleaning up our lifestyle act.

Antioxidant nutrients have been hailed as playing a major role in helping the body keep free radicals within safe bound-aries and in fighting against their negative effects. Studies have shown that groups who have a deficiency of antioxidant vitamins are more vulnerable to developing a significant level of degenerative disease than those who have a regular intake of these vitamins.

The Great Antioxidants

Antioxidants appear to act by fighting against the process of oxidation that goes on constantly in the body. The effects of oxidation can be graphically understood if we picture what happens when an apple is cut in half and left for a few hours. The cut surfaces exposed to the air develop a brown coating as a result of the apple reacting with the oxygen in the atmosphere. It is a similar degenerative process to the one that will inevitably happen if a car is left unprotected and exposed to the elements for long enough. Rust appears on the car, causing degeneration of its metal body – a parallel reaction to what occurs in the body as a consequence of unbridled free-radical production and the process of oxidation.

The good news for us is that the body has powerful allies at its disposal in the form of antioxidants which can help it minimise the damage from the inevitable process of oxidation. Since antioxidants are of such crucial importance, it is worth considering each one in turn, in order fully to understand their significant potential in supporting us in our experience of high-level health and vitality.

Vitamin A and Beta-carotene

The body has the capacity to convert beta-carotene into vitamin A, which is why beta-carotene is often referred to as a precursor to vitamin A. Beta-carotene is considered one of the most impressive and potent antioxidants because of its capacity to protect the cells of fruit and vegetables from shrivelling when exposed to the harmful rays of the sun. A deficiency of vitamin A makes us vulnerable to colds and flu, and to having poor-healing skin. Vitamin A also helps maintain the condition of the digestive tract, lungs and cell membranes, discouraging invaders from entering the body and viruses from gaining a foothold within cells.

A deficiency of vitamin A appears to have a negative effect on the thymus gland, causing it to become reduced in size, resulting in a less efficient and vigorous immune response. Reduced levels of vitamin A in the body has the undesirable effect of reduced antibody production, and a less efficient working of T-cells in fighting dangerous invaders.

OPTIMUM VITAMIN A AND BETA-CAROTENE INTAKE

Food sources of vitamin A are:

- oily fish
- liver
- eggs
- milk
- cheese
- butter

However, there are important practical advantages in choosing to supplement with beta-carotene rather than with vitamin A. The latter is fat-soluble and can be stored by the body, causing potentially toxic effects. This is why megadoses, either as food or supplements, taken each day are considered as potentially extremely hazardous: pregnant women, for instance, are advised to avoid liver and liver-rich foods because too much vitamin A can be harmful. Beta-carotene, on the other hand, is water-soluble, with the result that any that is surplus to the body's needs can be excreted.

Since free radicals are formed in plants a well as humans in response to exposure to ultra violet radiation from the sun, beta-carotene can play an important role in neutralizing the harmful effects of free radicals on sensitive skin. This essential antioxidant can also play a part in protecting average skin from the negative effects of strong sunlight, while also providing potentially anti-ageing effects when used in skin-care creams.

To have rich sources of beta-carotene in your diet, choose:

- fruit and vegetables that have a strongly deep orange or yellow colour such as carrots, mangoes or yellow peppers
- deep, dark-green vegetables: broccoli or fresh spinach are excellent choices
- parsley
- watercress
- asparagus
- tomatoes
- apricots
- peaches

As always, aim for at least five servings from any of these each day, brushing some of the vegetables with a little unrefined vegetable oil in order to maximize their absorption.

COOKING VITAMIN A AND BETA-CAROTENE FOODS

Cooking need not have a negative effect on beta-carotene as it tends to remain stable during cooking. In fact, some vegetables need to have their cell walls broken down by cooking before maximum amounts of beta-carotene can be released. With this in mind, chop, juice or purée regular helpings of fruit and vegetables rich in beta-carotene in order to encourage swift and easy uptake by the body.

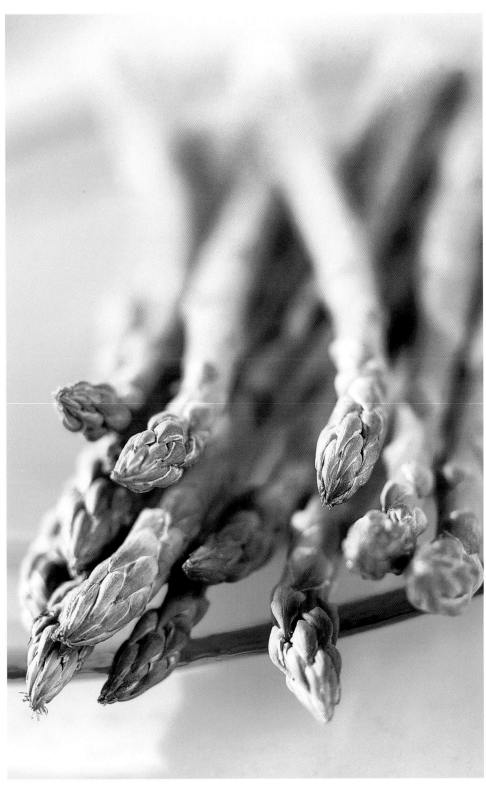

RECOMMENDED DAILY DOSES

It has been suggested that an optimum daily dose of vitamin A is around 5000 ius . The recommended daily dose of beta-carotene is approximately 7 mg.

Vitamin C

Vitamin C plays a vitally important role in helping the body fight bacterial and viral infections by supporting a vigorous and balanced working of the immune system. In addition, it plays a major part in promoting growth and repair of body tissues, as well as maintaining healthy skin and gums.

Vitamin C is one of the body's major antioxidant allies in helping fight the negative effect of free radicals. It is found in the fluid that flows between the cells, where it acts as a "search and destroy" weapon, effectively eliminating any free radicals that are unlucky enough to cross its path. It also appears to provide protection against viral infections by suppressing the process of virus replication and eliminating virus-infected cells. Studies have suggested that taking approximately 1,200 mg of vitamin C a day enhances T-cell activity.

Because vitamin C plays such a positive role in boosting immune-system functioning, we should make a point of ensuring that we have a regular intake of foods and drinks that are naturally high in vitamin C. These include:

- berry fruits such as blackcurrants and strawberries
- citrus fruits such as oranges, grapefruit and lemons
- kiwifruit
- parsley
- raw green and red peppers
- Brussels sprouts
- cauliflower

GETTING OPTIMUM AMOUNTS OF VITAMIN C

Unfortunately, vitamin C is a rather tricky vitamin to obtain on a daily basis, especially in the winter months when we tend to eat fewer fruits and vegetables. In addition, vitamin C is very readily oxidized when it is exposed to the air during preparation or cooking. Avoid chopping vegetables hours in advance of eating them to preserve their maximum vitamin C content.

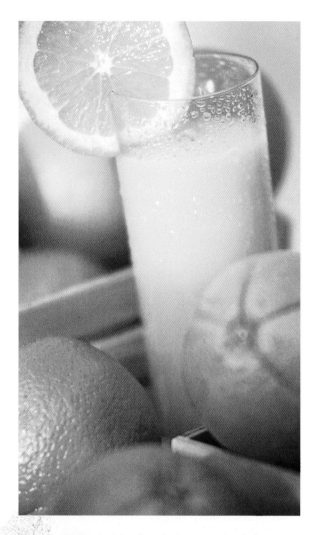

ABOVE: **Squeezing the juice from fresh oranges just before you want to drink it ensures it retains maximum vitamin C content.**

Make a point of buying fruit and vegetables in season whenever possible, since storing them for a long period of time has an adverse effect on their vitamin C content. For instance, potatoes freshly-dug in autumn yield approximately 30 mg of vitamin C; stored until spring, their vitamin C content drops to 8 mg. An exception to this problem is kiwi fruit, which retains most of its vitamin C content despite quite lengthy storage.

The way commercially prepared fruit juices are handled has a significant effect on their vitamin C content. If we keep an opened container of orange juice in the fridge for up to four days, the vitamin C content will have halved by the end of this period. We may naturally be inclined to shake a carton of fresh juice, but this is a generally bad idea as shaking promotes contact with oxygen (oxidization), which depletes the vitamin C content further.

COOKING VITAMIN C-RICH FOODS

Cooking vitamin C-rich foods appropriately is also important if optimum levels of the vitamin are to be preserved. The best methods is steaming; if boiling is necessary, make sure that the foods are plunged into water that is already simmering, rather than into cold water that will take some time to come to the boil. This is advantageous because the oxidizing enzymes that can attack and destroy vitamin C work less effectively at high temperatures. Soaking vegetables before cooking then putting them into cold water destroys a significant amount of their original vitamin C content, which leaches out into the water as it heats up.

It is important, too, to cook vitamin C-rich foods as quickly as possible, since it has been estimated that as much as 25 per cent of vitamin C can be lost after fifteen minutes of cooking, while a staggering 75 per cent will have been destroyed after cooking for one-and-a-half hours.

AMOUNTS TO TAKE

Because of vitamin C's water-soluble nature, the body can't store it for use in time of need, so we need to eat vitamin C-rich foods every day. The amount the body needs every day can vary, according to our experiences. Exposure to virulent viruses or bacteria, increased stress, heavy drinking, smoking, and taking conventional drugs can increase our need for vitamin C. Even being on the receiving end of a sudden, severe emotional shock can result in vitamin C levels being depleted.

If the immune system appears to be sluggish through the winter season, we should consider supplementing 1 gram of vitamin C a day as a preventative measure. If we have caught a cold, this dose may be increased temporarily to 2-3 grams a day until infection is over. If acidity of the stomach or slight diarrhoea develop the dose should be reduced until symptoms clear up.

Vitamin E

Vitamin E is regarded as an antioxidant of paramount importance because of its capacity to boost the immune system by strengthening white blood cells to fight infection. It also appears to play a particularly positive role in protecting the body against the steady decline in immune-system functioning that is regarded as being part and parcel of getting older.

Claims have also been made that vitamin E can play a vitally important part in protecting the health and resilience of the heart and circulatory system by discouraging LDL cholesterol from oxidizing and forming fatty plaques in the

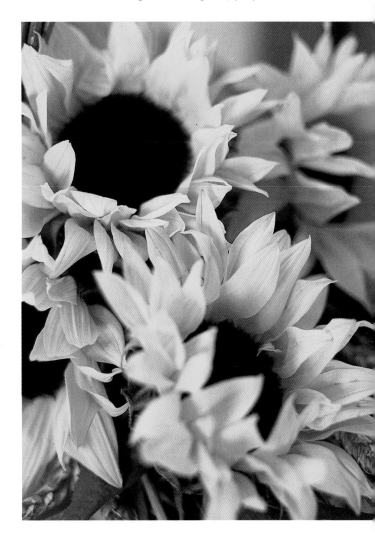

ABOVE: **Unrefined oil from sunflowers is an excellent source of the antioxidant vitamin E.**

arteries. This crucially important antioxidant also helps prevent any fat that we ingest from turning rancid in the body. This suggests that we should try to increase the amount of vitamin E that we take in proportion to the amount of polyunsaturated spreads that we eat.

As with many other nutrients, the beneficial action of vitamin E is enhanced by the presence of other nutrients, including vitamin C or selenium. This particularly applies to vitamin E's positive action as an eliminator of free radicals.

SOURCES OF VITAMIN E

Dietary sources of vitamin E are mainly unrefined vegetable oils including wheatgerm, safflower, and sunflower oils. Additional amounts may also be obtained from whole-grain products such as wholemeal bread and from nuts.

GETTING MAXIMUM VALUE FROM VITAMIN E

As with vitamin C, vitamin E reacts badly in response to certain cooking methods and storage conditions. Deep freezing and deep frying are particularly damaging: it has been estimated that the latter may destroy up to 90 per cent of a food's vitamin E content, a situation that can be made even worse if the cooking oil that is being used for deep frying has become rancid.

Storage needs care, too. The vitamin E in vegetable oils can be easily damaged through contact with oxygen, direct sunlight, or excessive warmth. Optimum storage conditions for unrefined vegetable oils are a cool, dark cupboard or the fridge, with the cap of the bottle always securely replaced.

AMOUNTS TO TAKE

Although a form of vitamin E is derived from a synthetic petrochemical source, an estimate has been made that this kind may be as much as 36 per cent less therapeutically effective than vitamin E obtained from a more natural source. To check whether a supplement is synthetic or natural vitamin E, look closely at the label. Vitamin E capsules from a natural source should include the letter "d" (d-alpha tocopherol), while a synthetic version will include the letters "dl" as a prefix (dl-alpha tocopherol).

A recommended daily dose of vitamin E is around 200 ius. Anyone who suffers from high blood pressure should avoid taking mega-doses of vitamin E as they may have a counter-productive effect. Instead, build up to a more conservative dosage slowly, acclimatizing the body by building up the dosage gently over an extended period of time.

Selenium

Selenium's role as a powerful antioxidant has been well established. It appears to provide significant protection against heart disease and cancer, while also providing an all-round immunity

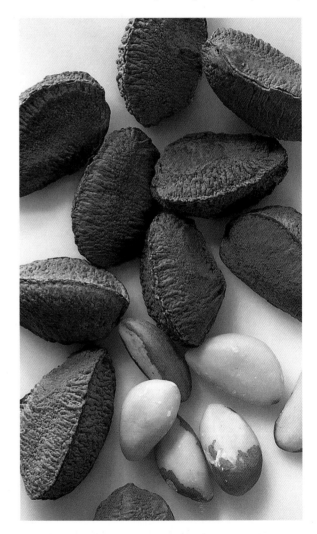

ABOVE: **The body's daily need for selenium can be satisfied by eating just one or two Brazil nuts.**

boost. This generally beneficial action appears to be linked to the way in which selenium, a mineral, is a very effective free radical scavenger, while also giving extra support in mobilizing T-cells and killer cells in fighting bacterial or viral infections.

Selenium also appears to play a significant role in helping maintain a healthy mental and emotional balance: studies conducted at Swansea University showed that people with adequate supplies of selenium have a reduced risk of anxiety, depression, or fatigue.

BEST SOURCE

Brazil nuts are an excellent dietary source of selenium: just one or two eaten each day provide the basic daily requirement. Eating the nuts is by far the best way of ensuring you get the selenium you need, because excessive doses in the form of supplements can have toxic effects.

Zinc

The mineral zinc is known as the thymus-boosting nutrient because of its capacity for supporting the working of this essentially important component of the immune system. Without a healthily working thymus gland, the T-cells cannot develop sufficiently to perform their important function of fighting threatening invaders.

If the body is suffering from a zinc deficiency it is likely to have a reduced number of T-cells, killer cells, and thymic hormone. Restoring zinc levels to their optimum condition gives macrophages a boost by eliminating undesirable invaders, while boosting the potential of the immune system to deal with bacterial infections.

People who are zinc deficient will have a generally weakened immune system response and a correspondingly increased susceptibility to recurrent infections. Certain groups have been identified as being particularly at risks of zinc deficiency. They include:

- People suffering from inflammatory bowel disease, which can lead to problems of malabsorption.
- The elderly, who tend to have smaller, less efficient thymus glands.

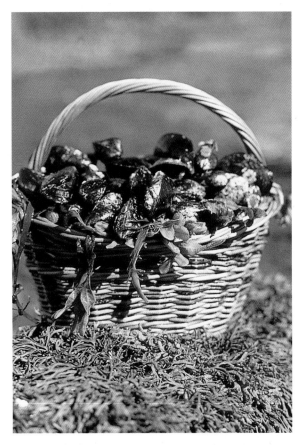

ABOVE: **Shellfish can help boost thymus-gland functioning. Always take care to avoid shellfish from polluted sources.**

- Alcoholics.
- Anyone who follows drastic eating plans or crash diets.
- Users of the contraceptive pill.
- People who take drugs intravenously.

GETTING THE BALANCE RIGHT

Zinc is easily obtained from foods. Dietary sources include:

- shellfish
- red meat
- nuts, especially pecans, brazil nuts, walnuts and almonds
- whole grains
- garlic
- potatoes
- beans

Aim for a zinc intake of approximately 15 mg a day. We might think that if zinc deficiency can cause such major problems with the proper functioning of the immune system, surely all we need to do is make sure that we top up with extra and our problems will automatically be solved. This is not the case. Taking too much of this essential mineral can cause problems by suppressing healthy functioning of the immune system. It is very important to strive for balanced zinc levels, best achieved by sticking to a daily maximum of 15 mg.

Co-Enzyme Q10

This antioxidant has been christened "the spark of life". It has a powerful immune-boosting effect which increases antibody production, and is an antiviral, antibacterial and antitumour agent.

It is a difficult nutrient to obtain from dietary sources alone, with the result that it is desirable to boost intake in supplement form. Possible dietary sources include oily fish, such as mackerel and sardines, offal and peanuts. A dose of approximately 30 mg per day is recommended for its immune-boosting effect.

Vitamin B6

The B-complex vitamins generally play a part in supporting the nervous system at times of stress, but vitamin B6 is also very much implicated in the work of balancing hormone levels, regulating prostaglandin formation, and supporting the immune system.

If the body does not have enough B6 at its disposal, the thymus gland will reduce in size and there will be a corresponding drop in the quantity of thymulin generated. The T-cells will not act as efficiently as they should, along with B-cell and antibody activity. Levels of interleukin-2 will also be negatively affected, and the consequent counterproductive effect on killer cells will leave the body vulnerable to infections or tumours.

Thus, it can be seen that a lack of vitamin B6 has a generally all-round disastrous effect on the immune system,

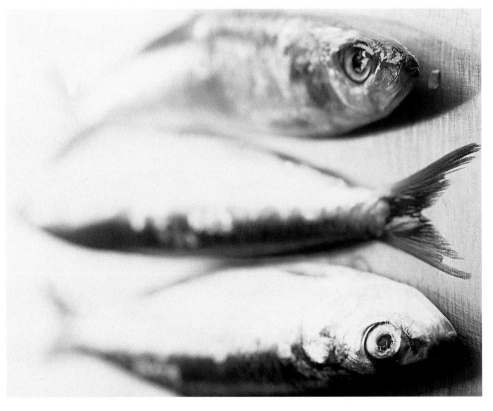

LEFT: **Making oily fish a regular part of the diet ensures good support for the immune system and for the health of the heart and the circulatory system.**

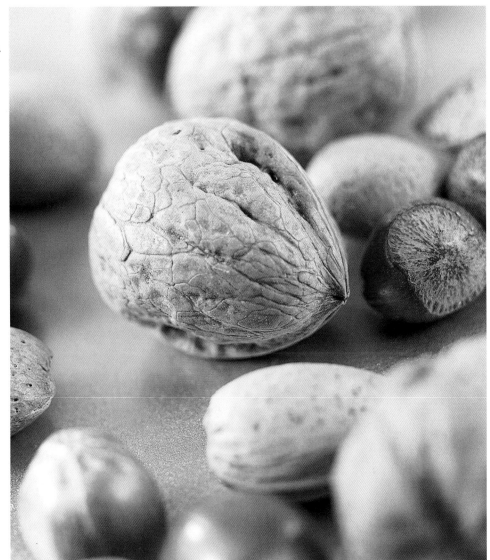

RIGHT: **Nuts and seeds are excellent sources of B vitamins as well as essential fatty acids.**

preventing it from performing as it needs to if we are to enjoy maximum health and vitality.

Vitamin B6 is best taken as part of the B-complex group of vitamins because they appear to work most harmoniously and efficiently when taken together. Special care needs to be taken with vitamin B6 as mega doses taken in isolation have been shown to give rise to undesirable neurological side-effects.

At times of severe stress, we would do well to consider supplementing dietary sources with a high-quality B-complex supplement until the stress has been resolved.

GOOD SOURCES

Dietary sources of B vitamins include a wide range of foods:

- fish
- poultry
- whole grains
- nuts and seeds
- soya beans
- red meat
- green leafy vegetables
- potatoes

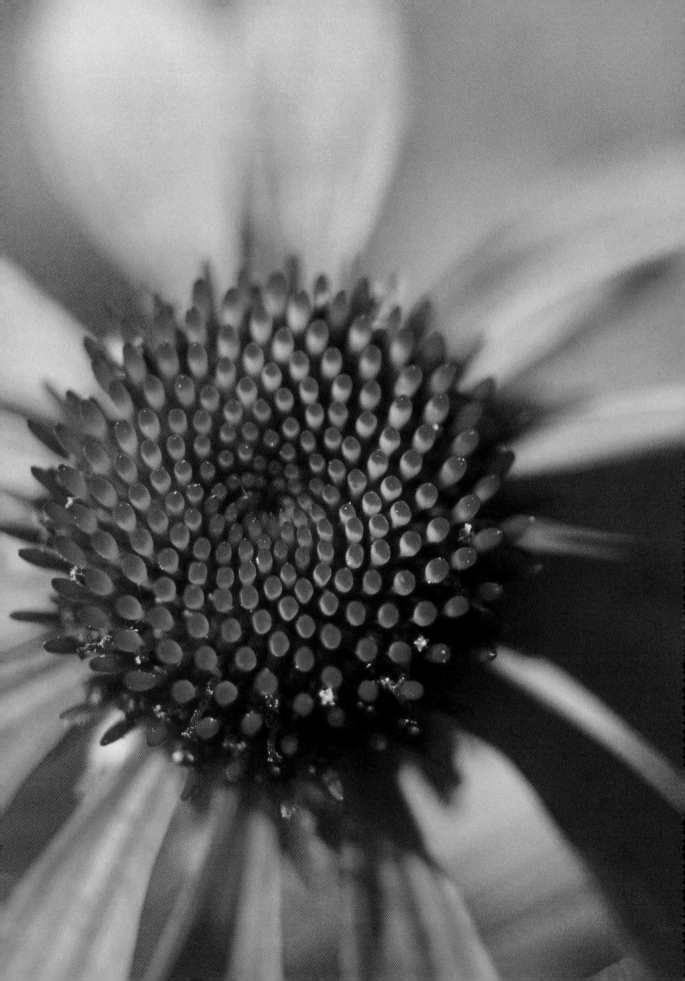

It is an extraordinarily empowering experience to discover the wealth of practical and effective support you have at your fingertips to treat a wide range of minor health problems. Although not serious in themselves, problems such as recurrent coughs and colds can do a great deal to undermine your general sense of well-being. In addition, constantly lurching from one minor infection to another can go a long way towards undermining your basic confidence in your body's ability to fight infection decisively and effectively.

Once you understand the practical measures you can use to boost the immune system's ability to deal with acute infections rapidly and efficiently, you will feel immensely liberated. Apart from anything else, you will be delighted to be freed from dependence on the routine, or too frequent, use of conventional medication such as painkillers and antibiotics.

The natural remedies for a wide variety of common complaints described in this chapter are free from known side-effects and are non-habit-forming. They also have an extremely impressive track record for restoring health gently, swiftly and efficiently.

Natural Treatments for Colds

Although hardly life-threatening, there is nothing quite like a severe bout of the common cold for making us feel absolutely wretched for days. Recurrent colds in the winter are one of the surest signs that the body is generally run down and at a low ebb.

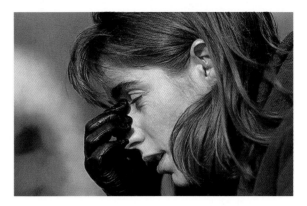

ABOVE: **The symptoms of the common cold can do a great deal to make the sufferer feel under par and sluggish.**

The biggest favour anyone suffering from recurring colds can do themselves is to take positive action, putting an immune system-boosting plan into action that is sure to give the symptoms of a cold their marching orders in double-quick time. These same measures will also go a long way towards protecting from any of the common complications of a cold, such as troublesome coughs, ear infections or sinusitis.

General Self-Help

- Rest as much as possible, especially in the early stage of a cold. However obvious and slightly boring this may sound, rest is your greatest basic ally in allowing energy to be used for fighting infection. If you insist in keeping on your feet, you are diverting this essential energy elsewhere.

Boosting 5 Immunity
with Natural Remedies

- Use natural methods to keep feverishness at bay, rather than using painkillers to suppress a moderately raised temperature. Drink fluids at regular intervals, opting for water or diluted fruit juices and avoiding tea or coffee, which are diuretic (fluid-eliminating) in nature and so will not keep up fluid levels.

- Don't force yourself to eat as usual if you don't feel like it. This will have the undesirable effect of raising your temperature and may make you feel queasy. Instead of eating a full meal, choose light, easily digested foods such as soups, broths and steamed vegetables.

- If your nose feels stuffed up and uncomfortably blocked, humidify the atmosphere of your room by placing bowls of water near each radiator. Alternatively, use a custom-made humidifier for the duration of your cold.

Essential Supplements

Two supplements, garlic and vitamin C, are essential weapons in the natural fight against colds.

GARLIC

Garlic has a powerful reputation as a natural anti-bacterial and anti-viral agent. As it can be difficult to eat enough garlic in its natural form to have a therapeutic effect, it is more practical and effective to take it in a concentrated form in an odourless tablet. The simplest way to take it is in a powerful one-a-day formula. For an additional boost for the immune system, choose a garlic supplement with added antioxidant vitamins A, C and E.

VITAMIN C

This vitamin is tremendously helpful in supporting the immune system in fighting infection. At the first sign of a sneeze, sniffle or slight sore throat take one gram of vitamin C a day. For maximum effectiveness, the supplement is best taken in a slow-release formula (500 milligrams taken morning and evening) so that it has the maximum opportunity for working over up to eight hours at a time. If there is any sign of indigestion or diarrhoea, reduce the dose until things have settled.

Herbal Help

Three herbs can be a great help in overcoming colds naturally.

ECHINACEA

A "must" if you want maximum support in getting over a cold as swiftly and efficiently as possible. Echinacea can be obtained in tincture, elixir or capsule form and should be taken according to the manufacturer's instructions for the duration of the cold. Above all, don't make the common mistake of continuing to take echinacea through the winter as a preventative measure as it has been suggested that the supplement has maximum effect when taken in short courses to fight infection.

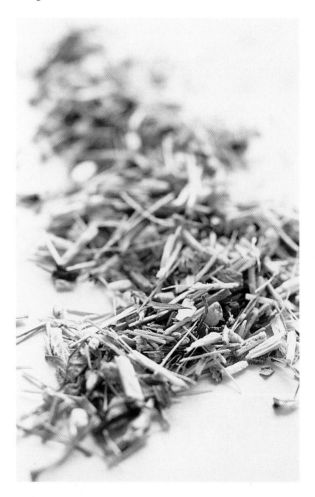

ABOVE: **Echinacea (also pictured on page 66) is one of the most effective immune system–boosting allies at our disposal.**

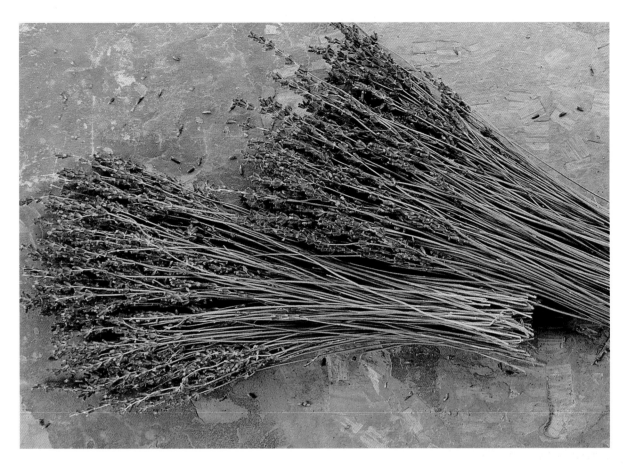

BASIL

A pleasant-tasting tea made from basil with a pinch of cloves added is soothing to an irritated throat and also encourages the production of a mild sweat.

ELDERBERRY EXTRACT

This has a powerful reputation for inhibiting the spread of viruses, and appears to be able to significantly shorten the duration of a heavy cold. It is available in lozenge or liquid form.

Aromatherapy

Several uses of essential oils are effective in helping reduce the symptoms of a cold:

- A few drops of eucalyptus, tea tree or lavender essential oil may be dropped on a tissue and inhaled whenever the nose feels blocked or the head feels stuffed up and muzzy.
- Blend four drops of any of the essential oils mentioned

ABOVE: **Lavender essential oil has powerful calming and mood-balancing properties.**

above into two teaspoons of carrier oil and massage into the chest or back as a soothing rub.

- Add five or six drops of lavender or tea tree oil to a warm bath for a comforting soak. This is best avoided if there is any sign of feverishness in order to avoid getting a chill.

Homeopathic Remedies

Choose from whichever of the following remedies matches your cold symptoms most closely. Once improvement sets in, stop taking the remedy since this is a sign it is doing its work and does not need repetition. Only recommence homeopathic treatment if the same symptoms occur as a result of a relapse, or if symptoms change. If the latter occurs, a new remedy needs to be selected that matches the changed symptoms.

ACONITE

This is a fast-acting remedy suitable for the initial stage of cold symptoms that develop abruptly after a chill or exposure to dry, cold winds. Symptoms may begin overnight or feel much worse when waking from interrupted sleep. There is a generally feverish state with sore eyes, nose and throat with scanty, clear discharges. The emotional state is very much affected when ill, leading to marked anxiety and restlessness that resemble the severity of panic attacks. Colds may also be brought on when the immune system is suppressed as a result of a severe emotional shock.

GELSEMIUM

This remedy is needed when symptoms develop slowly and insidiously over a few days. During this time, there is a

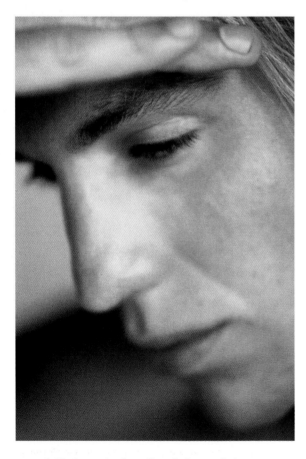

ABOVE: **Colds that make the sufferer feel generally hung over may respond well to the homeopathic remedy Nux vomica.**

characteristic sense of physical exhaustion, with heavy limbs, aches and pains and chills running up and down the spine. Headaches may set in with a sensation of a tight band around the forehead, with an unpleasantly blocked nose and swollen sore throat with loss of voice. There is a general sensation of being bruised all over with a tendency to be grouchy, bad-tempered and anti-social.

NUX VOMICA

This remedy is suitable for colds that cause a feeling of being completely "hung over" or cold symptoms that follow being run down as a result of working and playing too hard. Nasal passages feel much more uncomfortable for being indoors, and generally seem a lot freer of congestion in the fresh air. There is lots of violent sneezing with a raw, sore, itchy throat, and itchy ears. Headaches are severe with facial, neuralgic pain and queasiness. When this remedy is needed all that helps is peace and quiet and a sound, uninterrupted sleep.

NATRUM MUR

When this remedy is appropriate, there is a general state of feeling withdrawn and run down. Cold sores appear around the lips as a result of feeling low, and there may be a general state of low-grade dehydration leading to sore lips that crack in the middle. Nasal discharges alternate between running uncontrollably like a tap or being thick and clear like egg white. The emotional picture of this remedy is unmistakable, since there is a general desire to crawl away on one's own to recover, while any attempt at consolation and making a fuss is rejected.

PULSATILLA

Established cold symptoms respond best to this remedy, rather than symptoms that arise in the early stage of infection. Generally chilly, but feels much worse for being in stuffy, over-heated rooms. Nasal discharges are thick and greenish-yellow in colour, while catarrh is the same colour. The mouth feels dry without thirst, and the head feels muzzy and generally congested. The emotional state is very wobbly, weepy and in need of a sympathetic shoulder to cry on.

Natural Treatments for Burn-Out

This is a general state of emotional, physical and mental exhaustion that can follow on from an extended period of excessive stress, or the cumulative effect of a generally unhealthy lifestyle that is not giving the basic support needed to maintain optimum levels of health and vitality.

Symptoms of burn-out are wide-ranging, and may include any of the following:

- poor resistance to infections
- lack of concentration
- severe sense of physical and mental fatigue
- unpredictable mood swings
- unrefreshing or poor sleep patterns
- digestive problems such as acidity of the stomach, indigestion or alternation between diarrhoea and constipation
- inability to relax although feeling exhausted
- lack of confidence.

The advice offered below is most useful to people who are generally in good health, but who have found that a temporary crisis has left them feeling unusually wrung out and exhausted.

People for whom coping with stress is a long-term and well-established problem are likely to benefit greatly from professional advice to help them get to grips with this more chronic situation. Such support could initially be given by an alternative medical practitioner such as a homeopath, Western medical herbalist or traditional Chinese medical practitioner.

If you feel a psychological approach is going to be of additional help, you could consider seeing a stress counsellor or cognitive therapist. They are trained to help people gain a positive insight into the patterns that are leading to feelings of being burnt out. As a result, you should feel empowered to break the negative habits that are draining you.

General Self-Help

- Applying practical stress management techniques can be immensely helpful in preventing burn-out from taking

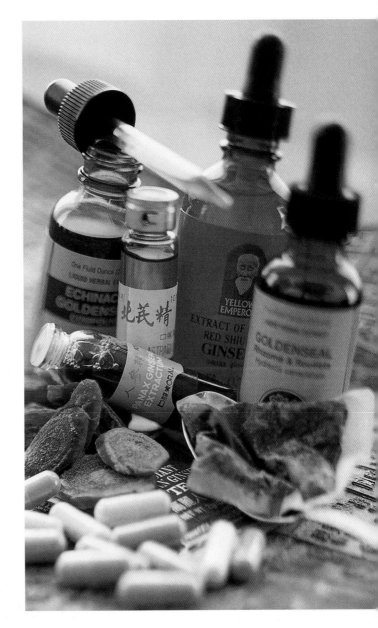

ABOVE: **Alternative therapies have important roles to play in treating stress-related symptoms.**

hold. One of the most basic positive strategies is making sure that however hard-pressed you may feel in your work, it is vitally important to take a break at lunch time. Taking a proper break has the two-fold advantage of allowing time for some relaxation and reflection and also allowing the digestion to work more efficiently and smoothly with what you are eating. There is nothing quite as likely to cause indigestion as gulping down a sandwich and a coffee while busily trying to concentrate on work.

- Make sure that you can turn down extra demands when you know you have reached your full capacity and any further commitments are going to be draining. Falling into the habit of pushing yourself beyond the point where you are functioning on a balanced, stimulating and productive level will almost certainly have you heading for burn out sooner or later. All that is needed to prevent this happening is to recognize the healthy boundaries you need to work within and make sure that you are not tempted or forced to move beyond them on more than a very short, infrequent or exceptional basis.
- Making relaxation techniques a basic part of your daily routine is one of the most positive ways you can keep burn out at bay. Enjoying regular, deep relaxation gives the mind, emotions and body a much-needed opportunity to rest and re-balance themselves. As we shall see in Chapter 7, "Boosting Immunity With Relaxation", the mind plays a profoundly important role in promoting a balanced and healthy immune system.
- An appropriate, regular exercise plan can also play a central role in keeping the mind, emotions, and body in balance, while also conditioning the immune system. When you are feeling stressed and anxious, practising dynamic but calming systems of movement such as T'ai chi or yoga can be invaluable in diffusing stress while benefiting the immune system at the same time. For more practical advice on the benefits of exercise see Chapter 6, "Boosting Immunity With Exercise".

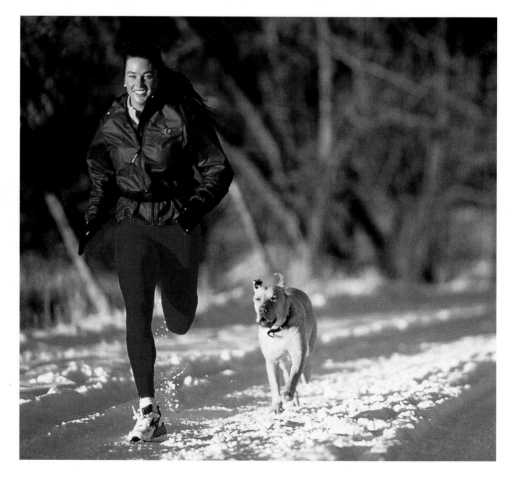

RIGHT: **Engaging in enjoyable regular exercise can to a great deal to reduce mental, emotional and physical stress.**

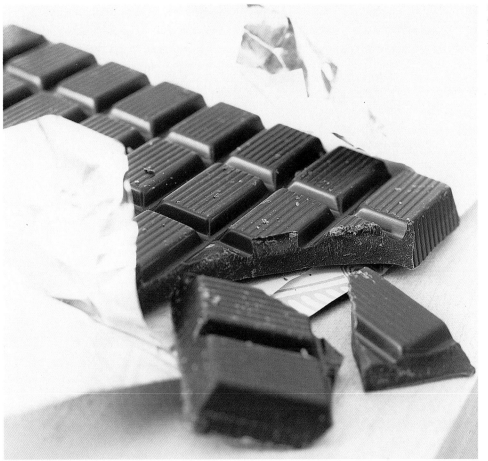

LEFT: **Chocolate contains caffeine, which can aggravate feelings of edginess and tenseness.**

- Bear in mind that what you eat and drink can help you avoid problems with burn-out, or make you more vulnerable to it. Foods that can contribute to feeling jittery, moody and on edge include sugary items, chocolate, "instant" snacks and any junk foods that are rich sources of chemical additives such as preservatives, colourings and artificial sweeteners. Drinks that can make you feel more burnt-out in the long run include strong coffee, tea, chocolate and alcohol.

Although you might think that the best way of giving energy levels a kick-start is to have a bar of chocolate or a cake and a coffee, the reverse is true. This sort of food or drink provides a short-lived, sharp energy boost rapidly followed by an equally abrupt energy slump as blood sugar is brought back to its cruising level. Once in this low blood sugar loop, you are likely instinctively to respond by taking more sweet food and caffeine in an effort to recapture what is doomed to be an increasingly short-lived energy rush.

This negative cycle can be effectively broken by substituting complex carbohydrates for simple carbohydrates. What this means in reality is avoiding sugary, refined foods such as sweet cakes and biscuits, in favour of wholemeal bread, organic rice cakes or a piece of fruit. Choose grain-based alternatives to coffee or have green tea, herbal or fruit teas when a warm drink is needed. Substitute sparkling mineral waters or carbonated, natural fruit-flavoured drinks for diet colas or other fizzy drinks that have a large proportion of chemical sweeteners or colourings added as well as a hefty proportion of refined sugar.

Essential Supplements

Three supplements, ginseng, schisandra and B vitamins, are particularly valuable in helping with the problems of burn-out.

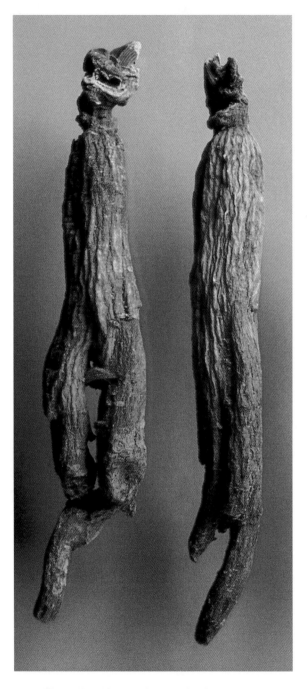

ABOVE: **Ginseng has adaptogenic properties that can support the body at times of stress.**

GINSENG

This has a well-established reputation as an energy- and vitality-stimulating tonic. Known as an adaptogen which is rich in saponins, it appears to have a powerful positive effect in stimulating the body to find a point of optimum mental, emotional and physical balance.

Ginseng has a history of use in the Far East going back 7000 years, and its positive benefits have been confirmed by clinical trials in our own time. These suggest that the positive action of ginseng is related to its capacity for supporting the body in adapting to physical and emotional stress and trauma. Much of the publicity surrounding the use of ginseng has focused on its purported aphrodisiac effects, but the positive effects of ginseng are by no means limited to this area. It appears that it also has stimulating effects on mental and physical energy, positively benefiting levels of stamina, concentration and resilience.

Ginseng also has a significant role to play in supporting the immune system, one study revealing that T-lymphocytes are found to multiply more efficiently in response to ginseng. Moderate doses appear to have a more beneficial effect in this regard than large ones, which appear to have an inhibiting effect on the immune system.

When buying ginseng, always choose the best quality available, rather than aiming to make a bargain purchase. This is important, since cheaper, inferior ginseng products may provide very little of the active ingredient.

The optimum suggested dose is 200mg a day taken in 100mg doses twice a day. It has been suggested that ginseng should not be taken on a routine, constant basis, but is best taken for two weeks, after which a gap of two weeks should be taken before beginning another course for two weeks. Ginseng is best avoided if there is any history of high blood pressure or cancer of the womb or breast.

SCHISANDRA

Schisandra has a great deal in common with ginseng as it is also rich in adaptogenic properties that can play an extremely positive role when the body is exposed to unusual amounts of stress. It appears to act by enhancing the uptake of oxygen

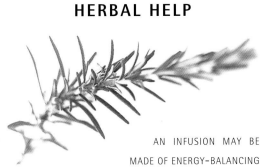
by the cells, and has been claimed to maximize concentration while also guarding against mood swings which may express themselves as irritability or anxious outbursts. The suggested dosage of 250–500mg may be taken in capsule form once a day.

VITAMIN B COMPLEX

B-complex vitamins can be especially valuable in supporting the nervous system at times of severe or protracted stress. It is important to choose a formula that gives the benefit of the full range of B vitamins because they are thought to work most effectively and beneficially when taken together.

Foods rich in B vitamins include yeast extract, wheat-germ, wholegrain cereals, seafood and green, leafy vegetables such as cabbage and Swiss chard.

Natural Treatment for Coughs

Although you may not think it while you have one, coughs are important allies in helping you get over a respiratory illness. Provided it is able to do its job properly, the coughing reflex is designed to help expel phlegm as it is coughed up, effectively clearing troublesome congestion from the chest. Once this has happened you should feel much better. The colour of the mucus, which can range from clear to yellow, green or brown, can indicate if a chest infection has set in (with a greenish colour indicating that it has). Provided a cough does not continue for an extended period of time without accomplishing anything, it should be seen as a vital support in

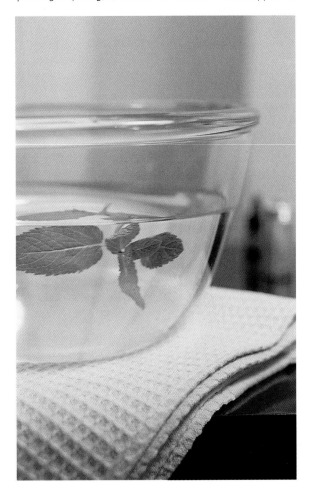

ABOVE: **Herbal infusions can have energizing or relaxing effects on the body, depending on the herbs selected.**

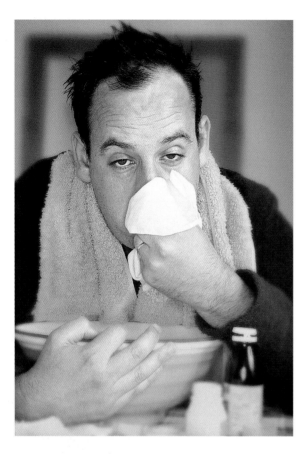

ABOVE: **Steam inhalations, with an appropriate aromatherapy oil added, if liked, can help clear air passages.**

General Self-Help

- If coughing bouts are especially severe or irritating at night, try sleeping propped up on two or three pillows. This can make you feel immediately more comfortable than sleeping lying flat as it allows the chest to relax and expand more easily.
- Coughs that sound dry and are irritating can be eased greatly by a steam treatment, especially if coughing bouts are aggravated by being exposed to dry, cold conditions. Try steam inhalations (using an appropriate addition of aromatherapy oils) or sitting in a steam-filled bathroom.
- Avoid the temptation to a have a milky drink before going to sleep, since cow's milk and dairy products made from it appear to contribute to excessive mucus production and general congestion of the nose, sinuses and chest. For the same reason avoid cheese, yoghurt and cream made from cow's milk.

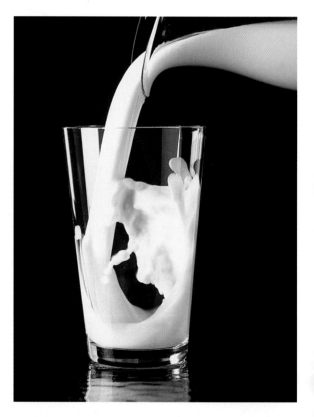

ABOVE: **People with colds should avoid drinking milk before bed, as cow's milk can contribute to excessive mucus production.**

helping rid the body of the toxic waste that is generated during illness.

It must be borne in mind that what is being talked about here is an uncomplicated cough that has set in following a cold or influenza. People with asthma, bronchitis or recurrent chest infections should seek professional medical help rather than try to handle the situation themselves.

When dealing with an acute episode of coughing in an otherwise healthy individual, an alternative medical approach concentrates on supporting the body in its efforts to break up and loosen phlegm from the chest. This is quite different from the conventional medical perspective which puts its efforts into temporarily suppressing the coughing reflex. This can have the unfortunate consequence of making the cough last longer and leaving the chest uncomfortably congested.

Essential Supplements

- Garlic when taken in a concentrated tablet form is an excellent anti-bacterial and anti-viral agent, while also encouraging the breaking up of congestive phlegm in the chest. One-a-day formulas are an excellent way of obtaining the therapeutic benefits of garlic with the minimum amount of fuss and disruption. If coughs are a frequent occurrence in the winter, consider taking garlic tablets as a preventative as the autumn sets in, continuing until spring.

- If a cough has set in as a complication of a heavy cold, see the advice on appropriate supplements given in "Natural Treatment for Colds" (pages 67-70).

Aromatherapy

Four drops of any of the essential oils tea tree, eucalyptus or sweet myrtle can be blended with two teaspoons of carrier oil and used as a soothing, aromatic rub to apply to the throat and chest three or four times a day.

Eucalyptus oil has head-clearing properties that are very welcome when we are suffering from congestive colds.

Herbal Help

- Dry coughs with muscular aching that arises as a result of the effort of coughing, may be soothed by making a mixture of honey and elecampane root. Use one cup of honey, one cup of water and a cup of elecampane root. Put the ingredients in a saucepan and bring slowly and carefully to the boil. Once the root has become soft, strain the cooled liquid into a glass bottle.
- Chesty coughs may respond well to an infusion of colts-foot, which is naturally high in vitamin C. Soak 25g (1oz) of the dried herb in 575ml (1 pint) of cold water. Bring the mixture to the boil in a saucepan, remove from the heat and leave to infuse for ten minutes. Strain into a clean container. Drink a cupful of the infusion three times a day until the cough has improved.
- If you don't want to make your own cough syrup, try two effective natural alternatives manufactured by the homeopathic pharmacy Weleda. These are cough syrups containing herbal and homeopathic ingredients. Palatable and pleasant to taste, the Cough Elixir is an excellent expectorant for chesty coughs, while dry, irritating coughs may respond more favourably to the Herb and Honey Elixir (see Useful Addresses, page 124).

Homeopathic Remedies

Choose from whichever of the following remedies matches your cough symptoms most closely. Once improvement sets in, stop taking the remedy, as this is a sign it is doing its work and does not need repetition. Only recommence homeopathic treatment if the same symptoms occur as a result of a relapse or if symptoms change. If the latter occurs, a new remedy that matches the changed symptoms must be selected.

BRYONIA

This remedy is immensely effective in clearing up dry, irritating, tickly coughs that seem to come from the upper chest. Confirmatory symptoms include painful, aching chest muscles as a result of the effort of constant, unproductive coughing bouts, also feeling headachy, bad-tempered and touchy as a result of coughing.

KALI BICH

When this remedy is indicated, there is a characteristic harsh, barking cough that is set off by a sense of irritation in the throat. There is great difficulty in bringing up mucus, which is stringy and ropy in appearance and texture. Coughing spasms are brought on by eating and by inhaling cold air.

PHOSPHORUS

Suitable for coughs that alternate between dry and loose in nature. Coughing bouts are brought on or made much more intense and distressing, by moving from one temperature to another. There is a characteristic tight sensation in the chest and some loss of voice with hoarseness or actual loss of voice with a cough. Mucus tends to be yellowish in colour.

PULSATILLA

Lingering coughs that are dry at night and productive in the morning with thick, yellowish-green phlegm may be eased a great deal by this remedy. Stuffy rooms and lying flat make the cough worse, while walking in the fresh air relieves it.

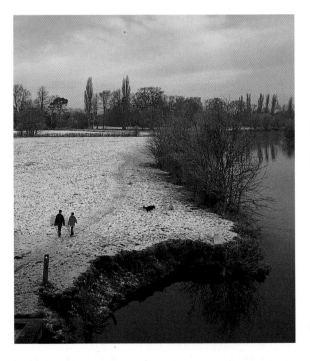

ABOVE: **Coughing spasms that are triggered by inhaling cold, crisp air, may be eased by the homeopathic remedy Kali bich.**

Natural Treatment for Cystitis

People are more vulnerable to bouts of this unpleasant, painful condition, which is much more common in women than in men, when they are run down, or during certain specific phases in life such as during the menopause or pregnancy.

If cystitis has become an established problem, with recurrent bouts occurring with depressing regularity, you need to seek professional medical advice in order to deal with whatever underlying factors are predisposing you to the problem. If conventional medical investigations and tests don't reveal anything positive or suggest useful remedies, you would do very well to seek alternative medical advice, which can be immensely helpful in supporting the body in fighting infection more effectively.

If, on the other hand, you are subject to very infrequent attacks of cystitis that tend to follow on from a period when you have become generally run down, the advice in this section may be enough to deal with the problem in the short term. Once the symptoms have cleared, you will be in a good position to get yourself back on track by following the general advice in this book on giving your whole system a needed immunity boost.

The common symptoms of cystitis are fairly unmistakable, and may include any combination of the following:

- an unpleasant, persistent bearing-down sensation in the lower abdomen which may extend to the back
- a constant urge to pass water, even when there is very little to pass
- stinging, burning or smarting sensations before, during, or after passing water
- a general sense of feeling ill, accompanied by a low-grade temperature
- strong-smelling, dark-coloured urine; in severe cases, urine may be cloudy and streaked with blood
- leakage of urine due to a sense of exaggerated urgency.

General Self-Help

- As with any other form of infection, deliberately taking it easy can help a great deal by liberating energy that can

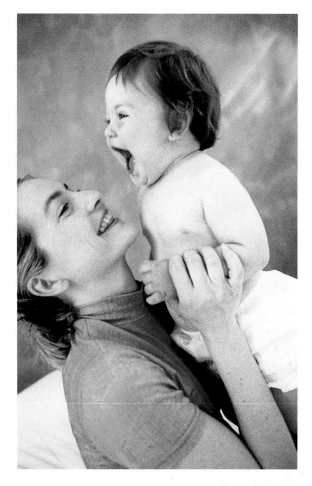

ABOVE: **Cystitis can be a troublesome problem during pregnancy or following childbirth.**

be used by the body to fight infection. This becomes even more important if you have a slight temperature or feel generally unwell.
- Avoiding getting a chill and keeping comfortably warm are especially important when dealing with cystitis as getting chilled can aggravate or bring on the problem, while warmth is generally very soothing and beneficial.
- If there is a tendency to develop cystitis it can be very helpful to get into the habit of never putting off passing water when the bladder is full since this can encourage problems to develop.
- Avoid wearing tight jeans, tights or leggings which create ideal conditions for bacterial or fungal infections to grow

Drinking cranberry juice
can help ease the distress
and discomfort of cystitis;
try to choose juices without
too much added sugar.

inside. Instead, wear underwear made from natural fibres like cotton and hold-up stockings in favour of tights.

- Drink lots of water and soothing fruit or herb teas to flush the bladder out. Avoid coffee and tea as they can make cystitis symptoms more intense. Apart from being irritants to the lining of the bladder, tea and coffee also act as diuretics, encouraging you to pass more liquid than you are taking in. Sugary foods and drinks are also best avoided during an attack of cystitis, since they can contribute to acidity.

Essential Supplements

Two supplements are very useful in fighting cystitis.

CRANBERRY JUICE

This has a powerful role to play in fighting cystitis. It can also generally reduce the incidence of urinary tract infections when taken on a regular basis as a preventative measure. This is thought to be due to an ingredient in cranberry juice which discourages infection-causing bacteria from taking hold in the bladder. Drink a glass of cranberry juice at the first indication of cystitis symptoms developing, making sure that plenty of water is also drunk in order to flush the bladder out fully. This should be repeated three of four times a day until symptoms ease. If cranberry juice is unappetizing, cranberry tablets are a useful alternative.

VITAMIN C

Taking half a gram (500 mgs) of vitamin C morning and evening for the duration of the problem can do a great deal to support the body in fighting infection. However, avoid taking citrus fruit as an extra source of vitamin C because of their irritant, acidic effects.

Herbal Help

- Drinking warm chamomile tea can be very soothing during a bout of cystitis. Apart from the soothing effects of any warm drink, chamomile has a specific reputation for easing muscular, cramping pains. The tea may be made from tea bags or by infusing half a teaspoonful of the dried flower heads in 300 ml (10 fl oz) hot water. Strain after three minutes and drink a large cup or mugful of this soothing tea three or four times a day until symptoms improve. This can be especially helpful if cystitis symptoms are made worse by

Chamomile has all-round soothing and calming properties.

feeling stressed or tense, since chamomile has a good reputation for soothing frayed nerves. Chamomile is also thought to support the action of phagocytes and thus boosts the immune system.

- Make your own barley water by adding two tablespoons of pearl barley to 1 litre (1¾ pints) of cold water in a saucepan. Bring to the boil, strain off the liquid into a glass bottle with a stopper or screw-top and store in the fridge. Drinking barley water (without the added sugar or sweeteners in commercially-made varieties) is very soothing during an attack of cystitis because it makes urine more alkaline and easier to pass.

Aromatherapy

Add a few drops of tea tree or lavender essential oil to a warm bath for a soothing soak. Alternatively, add three or four drops of essential oil to two teaspoons of carrier oil and massage over the abdomen to ease muscular aching and discomfort.

Homeopathic remedies

Choose from whichever of the following remedies matches your cystitis symptoms most closely. Once improvement sets in, stop taking the remedy since this is a sign it is doing its work and does not need repetition. Only recommence homeopathic treatment if the same symptoms occur as a result of

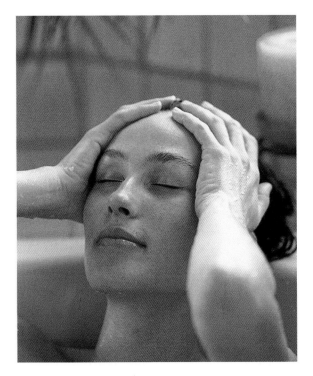

ABOVE: **Burning pains that are eased by warm bathing suggest that the homeopathic remedy Arsenium album may be helpful.**

a relapse, or if symptoms change. If the latter occurs, a new remedy that matches the changed symptoms will need to be selected.

CANTHARIS

One of the most commonly indicated remedies for easing symptoms of cystitis. Pains are scalding in nature and can occur before, during, or after passing water. There is a troublesome, perpetual desire to urinate, but only a few drops may be passed at a time. There is a general sensation of feverishness, shiveriness and chilliness when unwell.

ARSENICUM ALBUM

When this remedy is needed there is a characteristic burning sensation that is soothed by warmth: this could be provided by resting in bed, taking a warm bath, or putting a hot water bottle to the painful area. Symptoms feel much worse during the night, and there is likely to be a marked sense of physical, mental and emotional restlessness, as well as a strong sense of anxiety about being ill.

STAPHISAGRIA

A tendency to cystitis that has set in after childbirth or abdominal surgery may do very well with this remedy. Pains are stinging and burning, with a maddening sensation of a few drops of urine being left in the bladder that refuse to be passed. Cystitis may be brought on or made much worse for lovemaking. Extremely bad-tempered and irritable with the pains.

Natural Treatments for Sore Throats

Experiencing the symptoms of a sore throat is a sign that the body's first line of defence is doing its best in fighting infection. If this is a short-lived, infrequent, and not unduly distressing or disruptive experience, there is every chance that the body's defences are working well. In such a situation, the suggestions that appear below may do a great deal to get you over the episode of an inflamed and sore throat without any major complications.

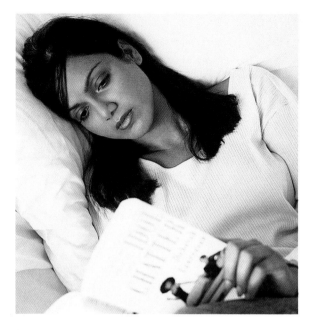

ABOVE: **Having an early night can do a great deal to speed up recovery from minor infectious illnesses.**

On the other hand, if you find that every winter you are plagued with one throat infection after another, you have a chronic problem that would be most effectively dealt with by professional, alternative medical help. Alternative medical therapies such as traditional Chinese medicine, homeopathy, or western medical herbalism concentrate on aiming to stimulate and support the body's own defences so that it becomes more resistant to infection as a result of effective treatment.

You should also experience additional benefits in the form of a general sense of increased well-being, greater vitality and improved emotional and physical resilience as a result of genuinely successful alternative medical treatment. This is due to the way in which the body's whole system is being treated and stimulated to work in a more balanced, harmonious and effective way, and not just the sore throat symptoms being treated in isolation on a temporary basis.

General self-help

- Try to avoid triggers that are known to stimulate the onset of a sore throat when resistance is at a temporary low. These include smoky atmospheres, having to project the voice for an extended period of time or having a run of late nights when feeling generally at a low physical ebb. Instead, make a deliberate effort to have a few early, restful nights, and make a conscious effort to relax. This need not involve anything elaborate: often staying in and reading or watching a video after a soothing bath may be enough to do the trick.

- At the first twinge of symptoms make a point of increasing fluid intake to keep your temperature from escalating and to encourage toxins to be flushed out of the body. Filtered or spring water is best; avoid citrus juices if there is a tendency to swollen glands as well as a sore throat. Avoid drinks that have a fluid-eliminating (diuretic) effect, such as tea and coffee, concentrating instead on soothing herb teas if a warm drink feels comforting. Don't forget that cooled herb or fruit teas can be flavoured with honey and spices and enjoyed as a long,

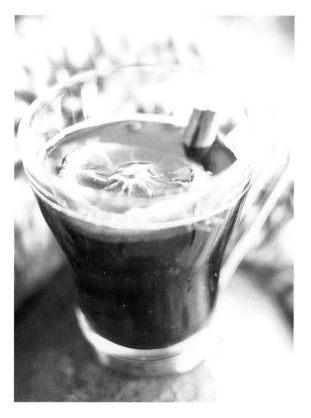

ABOVE: **Soothing, warm herb teas with added spices are an excellent and delicious alternative to a hot toddy.**

cool drink if they are prepared and then chilled in the fridge. These can be especially soothing to inflamed, sore throats that feel uncomfortably rough and dry.

- Inflamed throats also benefit from being lubricated by sucking soothing glycerine pastilles whenever the throat feel dry and uncomfortable. It is best to choose blackcurrant-flavoured pastilles rather than eucalyptus or menthol formulas when using homeopathic remedies. This is because certain strong flavours such as eucalyptus, menthol, or peppermint are thought to interfere with the medicinal action of homeopathic remedies.

Essential Supplements

- Increase the amount of vitamin C obtained from dietary sources, backed up with extra help from a slow-release vitamin C supplement, for the duration of the sore throat. Good natural sources include citrus fruit (except where glands are sensitive and painful), strawberries, blueberries, green leafy vegetables, tomatoes and raw peppers. This can be backed up by taking 1000mgs (one gram) each day, divided in two doses of 500 mgs, taken morning and

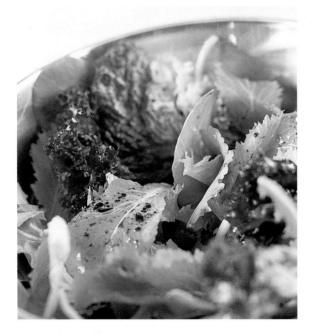

ABOVE: **Keeping the diet as light as possible can support you through the early stages of a sore throat or cold.**

evening. For severe sore throats, this dosage can be increased to up to 3 grams a day (divided into three doses through the day) until symptoms improve. Reduce the dose if diarrhoea or acidity of the stomach occur.

- The essential supplements suggested for colds (see page 68) may be helpful in dealing with a sore throat as quickly and efficiently as possible.

Herbal Help

- Grapefruit seed extract has been claimed to possess powerful antibiotic and anti-viral properties, and is thought to be especially appropriate in treating throat infections. It can be taken in tablet or liquid form. The extract may be taken two or three times daily as long as symptoms are causing a problem.
- Diluted tincture of hypericum and calendula can be used as an effective and soothing gargle for sore throats. The hypericum component of the tincture is a natural pain-reliever, while calendula is a natural anti-infective agent. Dilute one part of tincture in ten parts of boiled, cooled water and gargle as often as required.

Aromatherapy

Add three drops each of tea tree and eucalyptus essential oils to a teaspoon of carrier oil and gently massage the skin of the throat three or four times a day.

Homeopathic Remedies

Choose from whichever of the following matches your sore throat symptoms most closely. Once improvement sets in, stop taking the remedy as this is a sign it is doing its work and does not need repetition. Only recommence homeopathic treatment if the same symptoms occur as a result of a relapse or if symptoms change. If the latter occurs, a new remedy that matches the changed symptoms needs to be selected.

BELLADONNA

Early stages of sore throats that begin abruptly and severely with lots of throbbing pain and swelling, may ease considerably if this remedy is given early enough. There may be a craving for sharp, citrus-flavoured fruit drinks, but these may be very difficult to swallow because of severely swollen glands. The pains may be limited to, or noticeably worse on the right side.

LACHESIS

Left-sided sore throats that come on, or feel much worse when waking from sleep may respond very well to this remedy. Characteristic sensations include a marked sense of constriction in the throat that is extremely sensitive to warm drinks, and eased considerably by cool ones. There is also likely to be a marked aversion to wearing anything tight or restrictive around the neck, such as a scarf or neck-hugging jumper.

HEPAR SULPH

Sharp pains in the throat that feel as though a splinter or fish bone were sticking in to it, may improve greatly when taking this remedy. Glands in the neck are also likely to be swollen and sensitive in sympathy with the throat and pains are likely to have been established and around for a few days when this remedy is called for.

Natural Treatments for Thrush

Thrush is an unpleasant and irritating problem that can occur for a variety of reasons. Taking repeated courses of antibiotics in a desperate effort to get rid of recurrent infections such as cystitis can be one of the main triggers for the symptoms of thrush to arise. Antibiotics can have this effect because they can disturb the balance of the intestinal flora, encouraging Candida albicans (a yeast-like micro-organism) to spread beyond the confines of the gut where it normally lives quite happily. Once candida is allowed to proliferate in this unchecked way, it can give rise to the unmistakable signs of thrush.

This situation can be aggravated by additional factors such as a candida-aggravating diet (see overleaf), or by using toiletries that irritate the condition further. Thrush can also become a noticeable or recurrent problem during pregnancy or in people with diabetes.

The symptoms of thrush are fairly unmistakable, and may

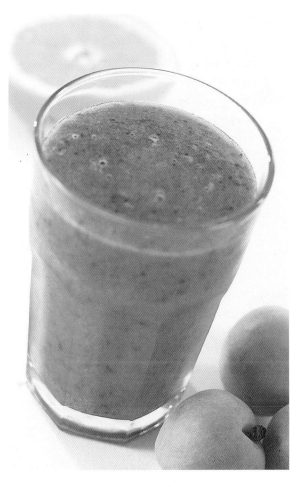

ABOVE: **Cool, freshly squeezed fruit juices can feel deliciously soothing to a rough, raw throat.**

include any combination of the following:

- itching and irritation of the genital area
- discomfort and sensitivity during love-making
- a thick, white discharge that looks rather like cottage cheese. It may also have a pungent, rather yeasty smell
- a tendency to want to pass water with greater frequency and/or urgency.

Apart from genital thrush symptoms, a general tendency to candida overgrowth may also give rise to a more general, diffuse series of symptoms that can have a negative effect on overall experience of health on a day-to-day basis. These can include any of the following problems:

- a pervading sense of exhaustion or persistent fatigue
- digestive uneasiness that may involve alternation between constipation and diarrhoea, bloating of the abdomen with excessive production of wind, acidity of the stomach or persistent indigestion
- joint pains
- mysterious skin rashes
- mood swings
- a tendency to low blood sugar levels
- fluid retention that may show itself in a periodical tendency to swelling or puffiness around the abdomen, ankles or fingers

If a general problem exists with an overgrowth of Candida albicans, it is important to seek professional help from an alternative medical practitioner to get to grips with the problem and rectify it at a fundamental level. If thrush is an infrequent problem that occurs in response to specific, known triggers, the following advice may be enough to deal with the acute problem speedily and effectively.

General Self-Help

It helps to be aware that there are specific foods that have a tendency to make candida overgrowth more of a problem. If you have experienced thrush on a persistent basis, or if you feel you may have a more general, low-grade problem with candida overgrowth, you would do well to avoid the following items as regular features of your diet:

- alcohol
- sugary foods and drinks
- cheeses
- vinegar and pickles
- mushrooms
- white bread
- tea
- non-organic red meat that is likely to have been treated with antibiotics and growth hormones

In other words, you need to be cautious about any food that is yeast-based, has refined sugar added to it or that has been subjected to a process of fermentation in its preparation. Foods you can enjoy, because they have a reputation for giving the body positive support in coping with candida proliferation, include:

- items made from whole, unrefined ingredients
- fish
- pulses
- raw vegetables
- brown rice
- natural live or bio yoghurt
- herb teas
- still mineral water

Natural live yoghurt can also be used as a local application to soothe irritated, sore tissue. Apart from the relief that is felt in response to its cooling nature, natural live yoghurt also appears to reduce vaginal pH levels by increasing natural lactobacilli levels.

Always avoid the temptation to use anaesthetic creams that have a short-term effect in soothing itching or irritation as all they are able to do is provide temporary relief at best. While this might seem initially desirable, the problem is that the cream is doing nothing to resolve the underlying imbalance that is leading to the symptoms of irritation and sensitivity. As a result, once the temporary effect has worn off you are

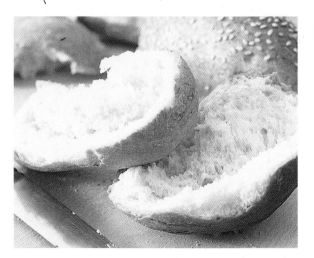

ABOVE: **White bread can be a health hazard because of the refined flour and yeasts used in making it.**

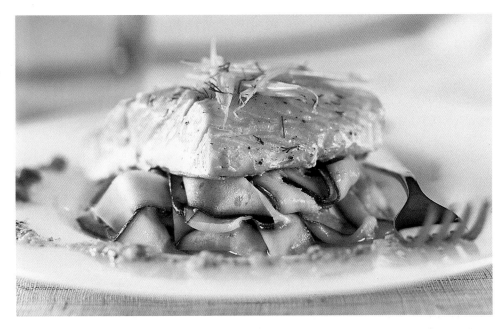

RIGHT: **When buying fresh salmon, choose organic or wild salmon in preference to the farmed variety.**

no further forward. In addition, creams of this kind can lead to further complications by encouraging the development of a sensitivity to the product when used over an extended period of time. As a result, you may not realize that increasing levels of irritation are being sparked off by a reaction to the cream, rather than being related to an intensification of the original problem with thrush.

If itching and irritation are especially severe, having a soak in a warm salt bath can be soothing. Add four table-spoonfuls of salt to the bathwater as the hot tap is running so that it has the best chance of dissolving and dispersing.

Essential Supplements

The following three supplements are especially useful:

GARLIC

As we already know, garlic has powerful antibiotic, anti-viral, and anti-fungal properties. These make it a major ally in helping the body deal with an acute episode of thrush. If the taste is appealing, add liberal amounts of fresh garlic to casseroles and soups, or use it baked as a tasty side dish. In addition, take a garlic supplement (ideally made from concentrated, powdered garlic) in a maximum-strength one-a-day formula.

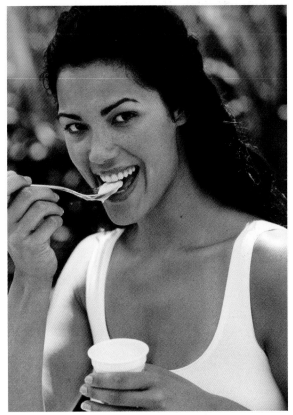

ABOVE: **Natural live yoghurt can play an important part in maintaining healthy functioning of the digestive tract.**

ACIDOPHILUS OR CAPRYLIC ACID

Recurring bouts of thrush that are due to a basic imbalance of intestinal flora may be eased by taking acidophilus or caprylic acid.

VITAMIN C

If a tendency to develop thrush occurs in response to emotional or physical stress or strain, you should consider basic immune system-boosting measures. You could begin by taking a daily dose of vitamin C to help kick-start your immune response again. Aim for a dose of 1 gram (1000 mg) initially, divided into two doses of 500 mg that may be taken morning and evening. While signs of the problem are still around, this may be increased to a dose of three grams a day, reducing the amount taken if digestive upsets occur.

Aromatherapy

- Use essential oils that have a reputation for helping the body fight fungal infections. Four drops of either tea tree, lavender or niaouli oil may be added to four teaspoons of carrier oil and used to massage the abdominal area and the back.
- Six to eight drops of tea tree oil may be added to the bath water to ease the discomfort of thrush, especially if it has occurred in addition to cystitis.

Herbal Help

- Herbs that have a reputation for possessing anti-fungal properties may be made into a strong infusion and added to the bath water in order to ease irritation and general discomfort. These include marigold, rosemary, fennel, or thyme. When making the infusion add a teaspoon of dried herb to a cup of boiling water. Leave to sit for fifteen minutes, then strain off the liquid and add when required to the bath water.
- Add an infusion of chamomile to a bidet and use it as a soothing wash for the genital area.
- Sip an infusion of blackberry leaf tea to help ease the irritation of thrush.
- If thrush has developed after a period of severe stress and

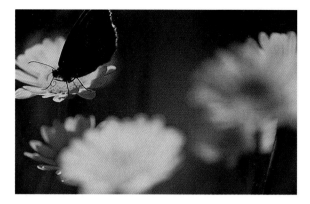

ABOVE: **Marigold has powerful anti-fungal properties and so makes a good herbal infusion for adding to a warm bath.**

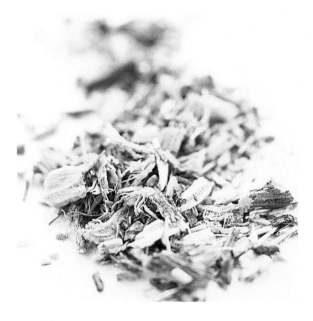

ABOVE: **Licorice helps the body bounce back after a protracted period of stress.**

it seems that the immune system has been compromised as a result, consider using licorice to help get the body's defences back on track. Licorice appears to have significant immune system-boosting properties, and may also play a positive role in improving its functions after a course of conventional medication such as antibiotics or steroids. It has also been suggested that licorice may play an important part in helping the body fight lingering fungal infections like thrush or viral infections such as cold sores.

Homeopathic Remedies

Choose from whichever of the following matches your thrush symptoms most closely. Once improvement sets in, stop taking the remedy as this is a sign it is doing its work and does not need repetition. Only recommence homeopathic treatment if the same symptoms occur as a result of a relapse or if symptoms change. If the latter occurs, a new remedy that matches the changed symptoms needs to be selected.

NATRUM MUR

When this remedy is needed there is a characteristic sense of persistent vaginal dryness with thrush. If there is a discharge it is likely to alternate between a thin watery liquid and a thicker discharge that looks rather like egg white. Despite the presence of this variable discharge, the sense of vaginal dryness is constant. Contact with warmth makes localized burning pains more intense, while cool bathing and cool compresses ease the general sense of discomfort.

BORAX

Episodes of thrush that have a tendency to develop at ovulation may do well with this remedy. Sensitivity and irritation are extreme, with an unpleasant and exaggerated sensation as though warm water is running down the thighs. There is a general over-sensitivity to touch, with symptoms either being at their peak mid-cycle or immediately following a period.

KALI CARB

This remedy should be considered whenever thrush symptoms cause a general sense of needing to pass water frequently and urgently. There is also likely to be a general sense of muscle cramping and discomfort, especially in the lower back area. Symptoms may be soothed by contact with warmth which counteracts a generally uncomfortable sense of chilliness, while they may be aggravated or brought on pre-menstrually.

PULSATILLA

Episodes of thrush that date from times of major hormonal upheaval such a puberty, pregnancy or the menopause may respond well to this remedy. Characteristic features include a

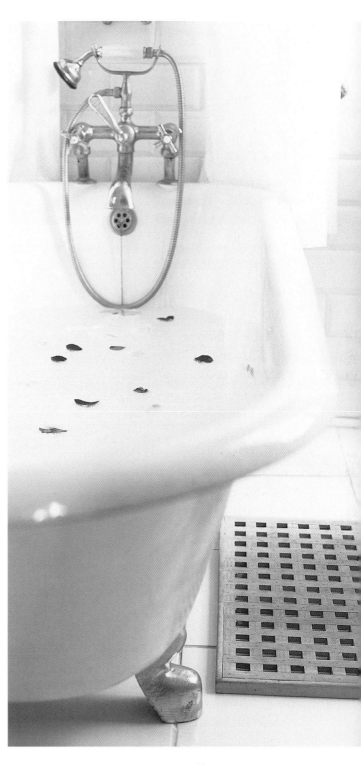

ABOVE: **A soothing salt bath can help ease the irritation and discomfort of a bout of thrush.**

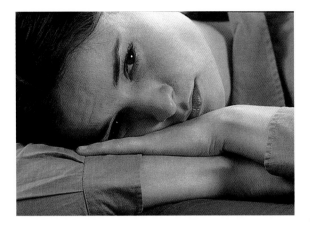

thick, bland, yellow-tinged discharge, with irritation that is made very much worse when getting warm. Thrush may be part of a general pre-menstrual picture, with a tendency to recurrent headaches, bloating and extreme mood swings with a tendency to be extremely weepy.

Natural Treatments for Digestive Upsets

A temporarily upset and generally disordered digestive system can occur for a variety of different reasons. Possible triggers can include any of the following:

- over-indulgence in an excessive amount of or an unfortunate mixture of rich food and/or alcohol
- eating contaminated food or drinking contaminated water (ice cubes are a common culprit for the latter)
- feeling severely anxious
- catching a bug that hits the digestive system hard at both ends, such as gastro-enteritis.

In addition, people may sometimes develop more long-term, well-established digestive problems that can set in in response to any of the following:

- an overly-stressful lifestyle which is not compensated for by developing skills in stress management
- a tendency to candida overgrowth

- a daily diet that is made up of items that are either hard to digest, or have a tendency to cause irritation or acidity of the digestive tract; these can vary from one person to another, depending on individual sensitivities and constitutional features, but common culprits include heavily sweetened foods, high-fat foods made from cows' milk, heavily spiced foods, deep-fried foods, excessive amounts of alcohol, coffee and tea and excessive smoking.

If digestive problems fall into the first category and have arisen out of a sudden, temporary digestive problem (for instance, as a bout of food poisoning), the suggestions below may do a great deal to get you over the problem as speedily and efficiently as possible.

If your condition falls more into the long-term category, you need to approach the problem from a more radical perspective. This often involves a fairly major re-evaluation of aspects of lifestyle that need improvement, so that having the support and guidance of an experienced alternative medical practitioner can be of immense value in getting you back on the right track. Even if this is the case, some of the advice given below is still likely to be of value and worth exploring as an initial step towards improvement.

General Self-Help

- If digestive upsets involve vomiting and/or diarrhoea it is vitally important to make sure that dehydration doesn't become an additional problem. To guard against this happening, drink as much water as possible. This is even more important if you have drunk too much alcohol, as hangovers are made doubly worse by dehydration due to the diuretic effects of alcohol. Avoid "morning after" headache and upset stomach formulas, since these contain painkillers such as aspirin that can lead to low-grade stomach bleeding. This is especially worrying because a tendency to bleeding of the stomach can be increased in the presence of alcohol.
- It's a good idea to start eating natural live yoghurt in an effort to re-balance disrupted intestinal flora. This can be of particular value after a severe bout of diarrhoea.

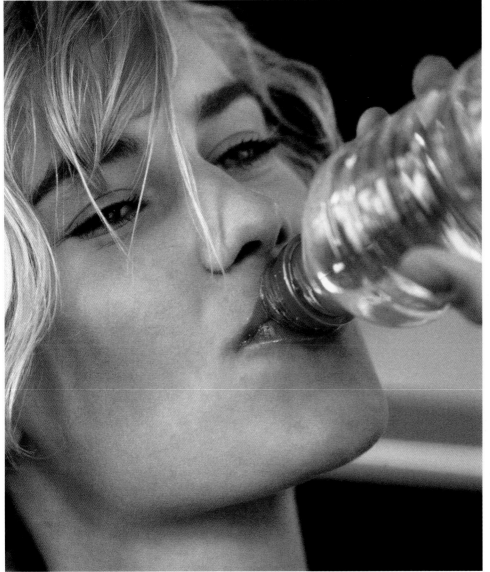

LEFT: **Avoid low-grade dehydration by making sure that five or six glasses of mineral water are drunk each day.**

- Certain combinations of foods that have a reputation for making matters worse are best avoided altogether when you feel queasy. These include red meat and potatoes, cheese with bread or sweet puddings with custard or cream. Instead, try fish or chicken with steamed vegetables or mixed salad, and fresh fruit in favour of puddings or cheese. Try a glass of freshly prepared carrot and celery juice or pineapple juice before a meal in order to stimulate effective working of digestive enzymes. Spices that are also thought to be digestive allies include cinnamon, coriander, cumin and cayenne (chilli).

- If indigestion or an acid stomach is an occasional problem, always resist the temptation to reach for an antacid as a short-term solution. There are specific drawbacks associated with routine use of antacids that can aggravate the situation even further. These can include raised blood pressure, or increased problems with fluid retention.

Cinnamon is one of
the spices that is
thought to aid digestion.

More insidiously, regular use of antacids can have the long-term effect of making indigestion worse. When the level of stomach acid is diluted after taking an antacid, there is a temporary easing of discomfort in the stomach. This favourable response is only short-lived, since the body responds by registering that levels of stomach acid have been considerably reduced. As a result, more acid is released into the stomach in an effort to re-balance the situation - and the situation is effectively back where it started, with burning and acidity in the stomach being experienced all over again.

If you are not conscious of what is going on, you are likely to interpret these signals as a sign that your indigestion has got worse, and your natural response is to reach for more antacids in an effort to gain short-term relief. However, once you understand how antacids can actually aggravate the situation, you will see that routinely taking them has the negative effect of making you dependent of medication in order to keep escalating symptoms temporarily at bay.

If there is an on-going tendency for the digestive system to function poorly, it can be of great practical help to make a point of regularizing eating patterns. Instead of leaving large gaps between meals and becoming ravenously hungry, when you are likely to be tempted to eat whatever is quickly to hand regardless of its nutritional value, you should aim instead to eat small meals based on nutritionally sound ingredients at regular intervals.

Essential Supplements

Two supplements are helpful:

ALOE VERA

This appears to have a powerful range of antiseptic and immune system-enhancing properties. As a result, it is thought to be especially effective in bolstering the body's defences when dealing with unwelcome stomach upsets and bugs. It can be taken in several different ways, depending on individual preferences. Tablets or liquid juice can be taken by mouth for digestive disturbances, while aloe vera gel can be applied to the skin as an effective cooling and anti-inflammatory agent in treating minor burns or irritation.

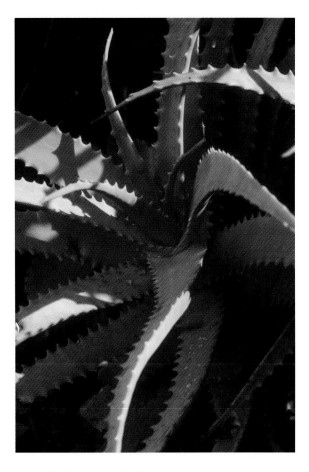

ABOVE: **Aloe Vera – an effective aid to the immune system.**

GRAPEFRUIT SEED EXTRACT

This extract has natural anti-viral and antibiotic properties which make it an excellent ally in helping fight stomach bugs. It may be taken in liquid or tablet form, depending on individual preference.

Aromatherapy

For general uneasiness and queasiness in the stomach, make up this massage combination and gently massage the area just above the rib cage with it: add two drops each of mandarin, ginger, peppermint, chamomile and black pepper essential oils to two teaspoons of carrier oil. Note: this massage oil should not be used for digestive upsets that occur during pregnancy.

Herbal Help

- Queasiness and digestive uneasiness that follow a wild night out may be eased by taking a few sips of any of the following soothing herb teas: fennel, peppermint or lemon balm.

- Ginger is one of the most effective spices for settling an uneasy stomach and has the added benefit of increasing the blood supply to the cells that support the immune system. If you are not worried about your sugar intake, sucking a piece of crystallized ginger is a delicious way of banishing queasiness. Alternatively, enjoy a sugar-free version of the same thing by making ginger tea. This can be made by infusing some freshly-grated ginger root in hot water, straining it and serving.

- Heartburn, acid indigestion, or general digestive uneasiness that follow eating an unwise combination of foods or too many rich ingredients, may be settled by taking a cup of slippery elm food as a soothing, warm drink. Slippery elm has a well-established reputation for reducing irritation of the stomach lining by providing a soothing coating. It comes in a fine powdered form, in malted or unmalted flavourings. Two teaspoons of the powder should be blended with a little warm milk or water to form a smooth paste. A cupful of hot milk or water may then be blended with the paste to make a palatable hot drink.

Homeopathic Remedies

Choose from whichever of the following matches your digestive upset symptoms most closely. Once improvement sets in, stop taking the remedy since this is a sign it is doing its work and does not need repetition. Only recommence homeopathic treatment if the same symptoms occur as a result of a relapse, or if symptoms change. If the latter occurs, a new remedy that matches the changed symptoms needs to be selected.

NUX VOMICA

This is the classic hangover remedy. Characteristic symptoms are unmistakable, and include nausea, constipation, severe headache and extreme irritability with an emotional "short fuse". Making an effort of any kind (moving, talking, or trying to concentrate on anything important) makes everything feel worse. All that helps is having a sound sleep in warm, peaceful surroundings.

PULSATILLA

Digestive problems that respond well to this remedy often develop after over-indulging in too many rich, fatty foods. There is likely to be an unpleasant sensation of a dry mouth without thirst with an upset stomach. Additional symptoms may include a tendency to frequent burping with "repeating" of the taste of the food that has set off the problem. If there is tenderness or discomfort in the stomach there is a good chance that it will be made worse, or brought on by jolting or jarring movements.

CARBO VEG

Severe indigestion with severe burping and flatulence will almost always respond well to this remedy. Characteristic symptoms include a disproportionate amount of bloating around the waist after eating even a small amount, with stuffy surroundings making the general sense of discomfort and uneasiness more intense.

ARSENICUM ALBUM

Food-poisoning symptoms that are set off after eating contaminated meat or fruit may be greatly eased by taking this remedy at the first signs of a problem. Characteristic features include vomiting and diarrhoea that occur together, with extreme distress and disgust at the thought, sight or smell of food. A general overwhelming sense of chilliness is likely to be present, as well as severe anxiety and physical and mental restlessness. Burning pains in the stomach may be temporarily soothed by frequent, small sips of warm drinks.

IPECAC

Awful nausea that is not relieved at all after vomiting, and made much worse by even the slightest movement may be eased by this remedy. Additional symptoms that would suggest this remedy may be helpful include colicky pains, distended stomach, and marked lack of thirst with vomiting.

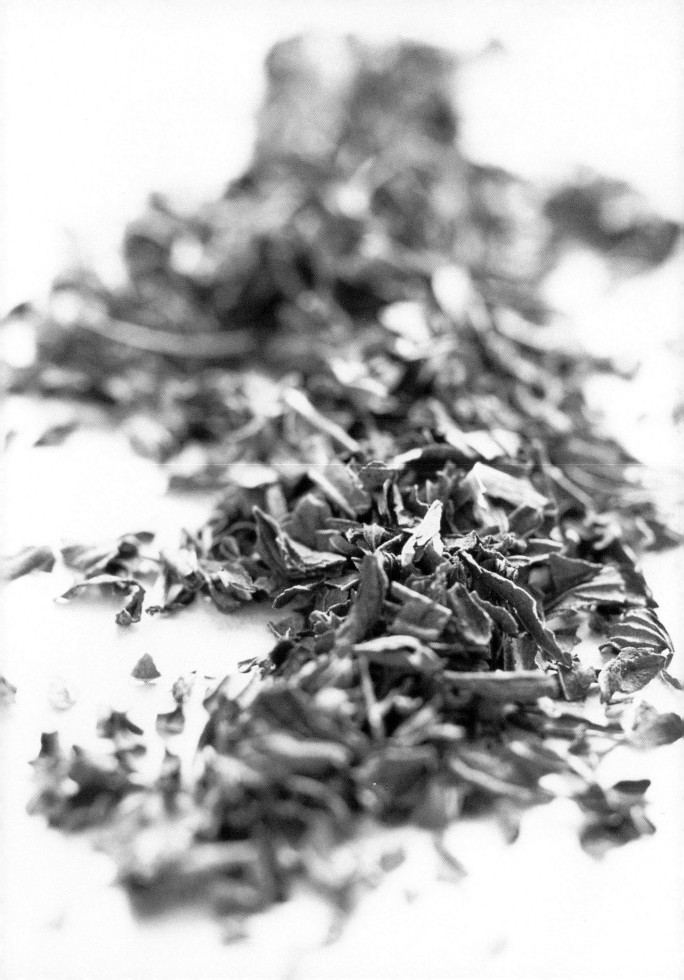

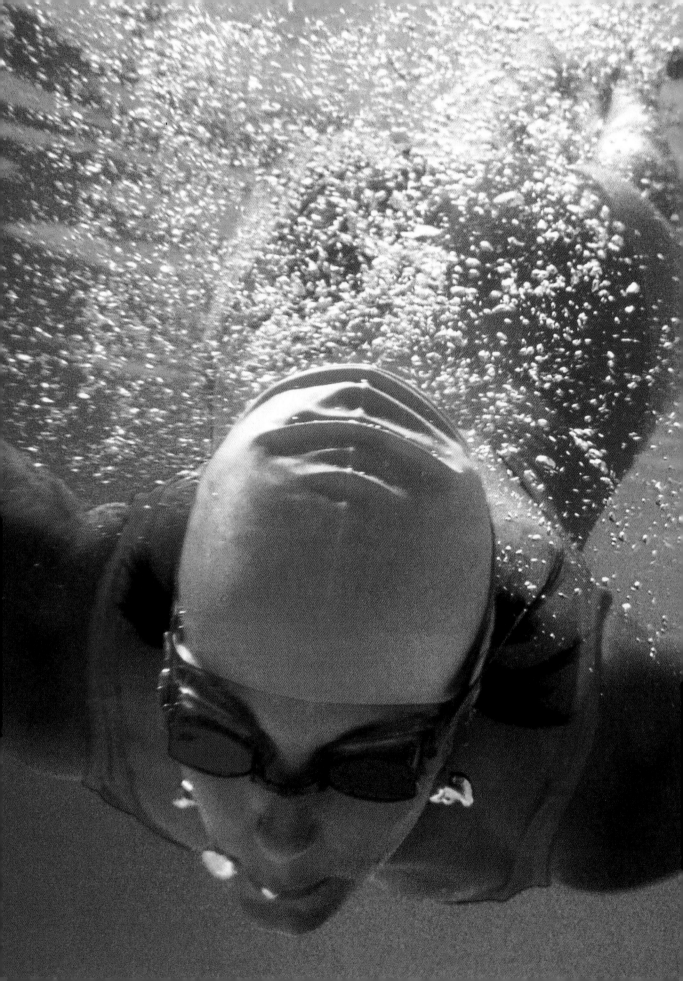

Most of us must by now be aware of the benefits of regular exercise. Over the past decade or two, much emphasis has been put on the need for us to take health-promoting improvements in our lifestyles very seriously. Many of us will be conscious of the links between an unhealthy diet, a sedentary lifestyle and an inability to cope with stress and a whole host of degenerative diseases such as heart disease, diabetes and stroke.

It has been estimated that even for people who have been unfit in their youth, taking up a balanced exercise programme in their middle years can reduce the risk of developing the conditions listed above by as much as 40 per cent. In addition, regular exercise may mean reducing the risk of developing cancer of the colon, rectum and womb by as much as 25 per cent. If this is the case, just imagine how significant the health benefits must be if regular exercise is combined with a nutritious diet and a good stress-management plan.

It is important to emphasize that what should be aimed for is a balanced regime of physical activity that avoids the pitfalls of over-training. This is especially important if the immune system is to be boosted, since a too-vigorous exercise programme appears to have a negative effect by temporarily suppressing the immune system.

As in so many aspects of looking after our health, achieving a healthy, optimum state of balance appears to be the key, rather than being seduced by an extreme or drastic approach. This is something that those who tend towards short-cuts to health and fitness should always bear in mind, since expecting to turn the fitness tables around too abruptly after years of physical inactivity may do more harm than good.

Taking Control

Once we begin to make exercise a regular part of our lives, we are likely to develop a very positive feeling that we are not slaves to bodies that are programmed to become sick and less resilient, and may begin to enjoy the empowering sensation that we are able to take positive steps to support and protect our body's self-healing mechanism. Feeling we are in the driving seat can do an enormous amount to build up our sense of confidence in our body, which in itself can contribute to our enjoying better quality health.

Our thoughts can become self-fulfilling: if we see ourselves as frail and helpless, there is a good chance that this is what we will become and how others will view us. If we feel positive, confident in our body and strong, there is an equally fighting chance that this is what we will become in our own eyes, and in other people's, too.

Taking regular exercise can contribute an enormous amount to this process. It boosts the performance of the

Boosting Immunity

with Exercise &
Body-Conditioning Techniques

immune system, helps to provide an essential outlet for stress, and makes the body stronger, leaner, more flexible and more resilient. Everything in this chapter is aimed at helping you understand how appropriate exercise and basic body maintenance has a positive impact on the body's defences, and how you can set about getting moving if you have previously considered yourself unfit.

Exercise and the Immune System

The body is dependent on the efficient flow of lymphatic fluid to help eliminate toxins from its systems. When the body's immune system is functioning smoothly, the lymphatic system, which includes the lymph nodes that are found in the neck, armpits and groin, are likely to be working at peak efficiency. When the immune system is working vigorously, toxins and dead cells are swept along by the lymphatic fluid in the lymphatic vessels to the lymph nodes, whose job is to eliminate any impurities before the fluid is directed back to the bloodstream.

Unlike the circulatory system, which has the powerful pumping power of the heart and arterial pressure to keep it moving, the lymphatic system has no such organ to help guard against undesirable stagnation. Instead, it is dependent on the muscular contractions of the main muscle groups, or the force of gravity to keep the lymphatic fluid on the move.

A sedentary lifestyle, in which the muscles in the legs and arms are not moving regularly, can encourage stagnation of the circulation and lymphatic fluid. If this goes on for an extended period of time, it can be a significant contributing factor to problems with persistent fatigue and generally poor elimination of toxins from the body.

On the other hand, if you get moving and enjoy exercise that contracts and expands the major muscles in your arms and legs, you are giving your lymphatic system the boost needed to work more efficiently. As a result, you should feel more energized, stronger and more resilient in fighting low-grade infections.

An additional cosmetic benefit of encouraging more efficient drainage of lymphatic fluid is cellulite reduction. This is

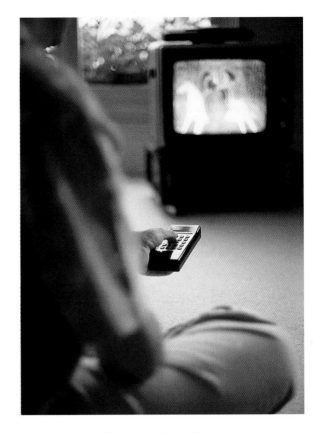

ABOVE: **A sedentary lifestyle can be a major contributory factor in making you feel sluggish and fatigued.**

a controversial issue, with some medical specialists suggesting that cellulite doesn't really exist. Those who view health issues from a more holistic perspective see the presence of cellulite as a basic indicator of sluggish, inefficient lymphatic and circulatory systems. From this point of view, it makes a great deal of sense to monitor the amount of cellulite on the body as a basic indicator of how well or not it is eliminating toxins. There is detailed advice on setting about effective cellulite reduction in the sections on body brushing and hydrotherapy techniques below (see pages 108-110).

Exercise and Emotional Balance

The negative effect that unmanageable stress can have on the immune system is explored in detail in the following chapter. However, it is relevant to spend a little time at this point

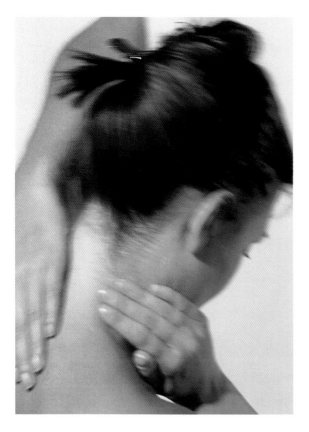

ABOVE: **People who suffer from recurrent tension headaches may benefit greatly from regular neck and shoulder massage.**

that gets progressively more severe. Fortunately, there are important practical tools at our disposal for turning this negative pattern of stress response into a positive pattern of stress reduction and effective management. Two of the most important tools are appropriate, regular exercise and relaxation techniques. The latter are explored in the next chapter, with additional stress-management strategies.

Appropriate physical activity plays a profoundly significant role in helping diffuse stress. This is because non-competitive systems of exercise which combine awareness of movement with relaxation techniques, such as yoga (see page 104) or t'ai chi (see page 105), put you in touch with areas of tension in the body. Once you have developed this awareness, you are in an excellent position to be able to consciously relax tight muscle groups. Although not strictly considered an exercise system, the Alexander Technique (see page 107) can be especially valuable in helping you develop an awareness of areas of your body where you are holding tension.

In addition, forms of exercise that include deep stretching movements, such as yoga, t'ai chi, or Pilates (see page 104) allow you to release tension from tight, bunched-up muscle groups, while at the same time developing a formidable sense of muscle strength, stamina and suppleness. It has also been suggested that the "Yogacise" method of yoga may also improve cellulite by promoting deep-stretching exercises that help elongate muscles, making them generally leaner, as well as discouraging the production of cellulite.

considering the important benefits that appropriate exercise can bring to the body's ability to manage stress and, as a result, to contribute to an enhanced sense of emotional equilibrium.

When we feel stressed, we tend to tense our muscles generally, and particularly those of the neck, shoulders, upper arms and back. This general state of muscular tension, if it goes on long enough, will contribute to the production of tension headaches, back pain, poor sleep patterns and a host of digestive problems. If such physical symptoms persist, they are likely to cause even more stress and lead to a vicious circle of emotional, mental and physical tension

Regular exercise puts us in touch with our bodies, helping us identify weak areas.

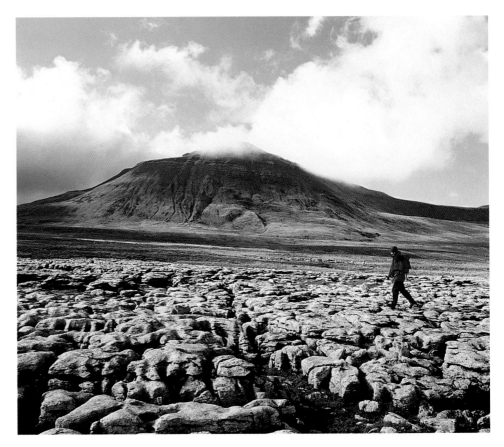

RIGHT: **Walking is one of the most beneficial forms of aerobic exercise readily available to us.**

It has also been suggested that regular aerobic exercise, such as brisk walking or cycling, that conditions the heart and lungs can play an important role in helping counteract negative emotions such as depression. It may also assist those who suffer from chronic anxiety to calm down considerably and experience a much more balanced and tranquil state of mind. This appears to be due to the way in which regular, rhythmical aerobic exercise promotes the secretion of chemicals in the body called endorphins. These have natural anti-depressant and pain-relieving properties, and are responsible for the "high" that follows vigorous, but not excessively challenging exercise.

Since a positive state of mind appears to have a significant impact on the functioning and condition of the immune system, this mood-balancing, "feel good" aspect of regular exercise is an important element to consider in any programme aimed at boosting the functioning of the immune system with natural methods.

What is perhaps most significant about the direction that exercise is currently taking is the way in which the emphasis is falling naturally on non-competitive systems, such as the ones mentioned above. This is an extremely positive development from the point of view of stress-management and immune system support as indulging in an overly-taxing exercise regime for example training for marathons can lead to increased stress levels, a depressed immune system and possible problems with exercise addiction.

If you take a non-competitive approach, making exercise a regular, enjoyable and relaxing part of your life, you should find that you enable yourself to make your life more balanced rather than causing yourself greater stress and pressure. Once you have achieved this sense of basic balance you should find that your energy levels are boosted, you have greater resistance to minor infection and you generally feel more relaxed and emotionally, mentally and physically resilient.

Basic Guidelines for Getting Physically Fit

Many of us may have been put off exercising by being too ambitious and setting unrealistic goals. We may have been unable to make the necessary time available to go to the gym, may have started a too-demanding training programme, or chosen a range of exercise activities that were boring, but which we followed because they were the trendiest health kick at the time.

These are extremely common mistakes made by many would-be exercisers, especially if they were converted to exercise in the 1980s with its obsession with physical competitiveness and its mantras of "going for the burn" or "no pain, no gain". By the early 1990s it was already becoming uncomfortably clear that the punishing jogging programmes and aerobics classes of the preceding decade had left behind a less than healthy legacy. Too many people had injured knees, ankles and backs as a result of an overly competitive and punishing approach to physical fitness.

Thankfully, a fresh perspective on exercise developed through the 1990s that was more in keeping with the general move towards a holistic approach to health. As a result, we began to see that little would be gained in the health stakes from treating our bodies as machines that could take any amount of pain or punishing, stress-inducing physical exertion. Instead, we began to see our bodies as being part of a complex interaction between emotions, mind and physical experience. The emphasis also changed from competitiveness and disciplining the body to a more positive search for balance and harmony.

Perhaps most significantly of all, we began to appreciate that each of us is an unique individual with our own strengths and limitations. Whatever system of physical activity we might choose, it would need to fit our very special individual requirements, constitutions and temperaments if we are to have the best chance of enjoying the potential benefits that an appropriate exercise programme can bring.

RIGHT: **For exercise to be truly beneficial, it must be appropriate to the exerciser's temperament and physical capabilities.**

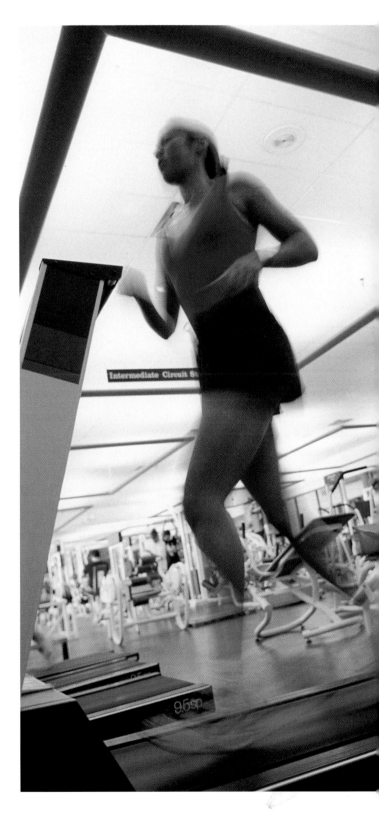

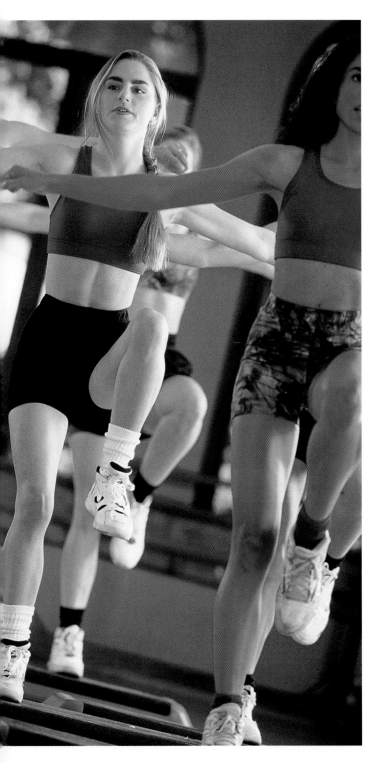

Choosing an Exercise Programme

Follow this general advice and you will bypass the common mistakes that many people make when they decide to set about getting physically fit.

- Always ensure that the programme of exercise you choose is going to be fun and enjoyable. You are unlikely to be motivated to keep on doing something you find boring or unenjoyable.

- Assess carefully your own unique requirements, tastes and preferences. These must be met if any programme of physical fitness is going to match your emotional, mental and physical needs.

- Consider carefully how fit you are already and make sure that whatever activity you choose is appropriate for the level you are starting from. Above all, always avoid the temptation to dive in at the deep end: it is far better to build your fitness level slowly and steadily, to avoid putting undue strain on your body.

- Always be ruthlessly realistic about the time you can devote to exercising. If a fitness programme is to be successful, you must be sure from the beginning that you can support on a long-term basis the amount of time you are proposing to spend in exercise. The secret of succeeding is being deliberately modest rather than overly-ambitious when assessing how much time you have to spare.

- Always bear in mind that once you have made a solid start, you are likely to be feeling so motivated by the benefits you are seeing that you will have the enthusiasm to make more time available. You will be allowing a more demanding exercise schedule to develop in a natural and organic way so that the habit has the best chance of continuing. Making the common mistake of putting yourself under unrealistic and unachievable pressure at the beginning is all too likely to result in your giving up rapidly, however well-intentioned you were at the outset.

- If you have a failed fitness experience behind you, consider how suited your choice of fitness activity was to your temperament. This time, don't automatically

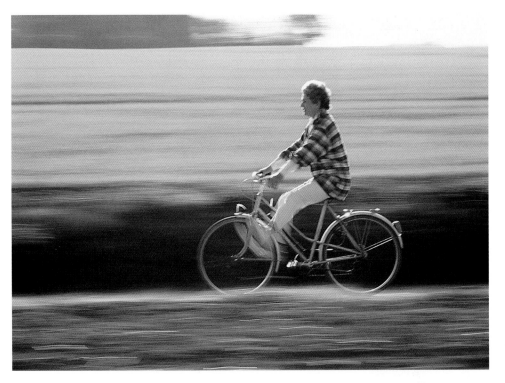

choose the obvious, but let your imagination wander and you might be surprised at the possibilities you have overlooked in the past.

- Work out what your fitness priorities are, and choose a programme of physical fitness activities that will help work on those areas.

The lists that follow cover those areas of the body that most commonly need attention among people who have not been in the habit of exercising regularly, with suggestions for the forms of exercise systems that may best benefit them.

POOR MUSCLE STRENGTH AND MUSCLE TONE

- Swimming
- Aqua aerobics
- Weight training
- Pilates
- Body sculpting
- Yoga
- Power walking

LACK OF AEROBIC FITNESS

- Cycling
- Swimming
- Skipping
- Brisk walking
- Running
- Dancing
- Step aerobics

POOR GENERAL FLEXIBILITY

- Yoga
- T'ai chi
- Pilates
- Stretch and tone classes

PROBLEMS WITH TENSE, UNRELAXED MUSCLES

- Alexander technique
- Autogenic training
- Yoga
- T'ai chi
- Qi gong
- Regular practice of relaxation techniques

Special Exercise Techniques and Therapies

Some of the activities mentioned above, such as swimming, walking, cycling and skipping, are self-explanatory. Others may be less familiar. What follows are concise descriptions of some of the less common, but very beneficial, forms of exercise. Relaxation techniques are described in "Boosting Immunity With Relaxation" (page 112).

Yoga

Many of us know that yoga is a centuries-old system of exercise, but we may not be aware of how perfectly it fits with the twenty-first century ideal model of integrated physical and mental fitness. Yoga provides a system of movement that allows for the ultimate conditioning of the body, while also encouraging relaxation and balance of the mind.

Practising yoga regularly is a non-competitive way of building exceptional muscular strength, stamina and flexibility, while also teaching basic breathing skills that induce a state of mental and emotional tranquillity and harmony.

Yoga is an especially attractive option for those who may have been turned off by competitive, macho sports as a child. If you are such a person, you will be delighted to discover that when you practise yoga, you are in competition with no one but yourself. You should never find that you have to push yourself beyond physical boundaries that cause discomfort.

Pilates

This system of exercise has become increasingly popular over the past decade. Originally developed in the 1920s as a physiotherapeutic system, the Pilates approach to exercise concentrates on the participant developing a keen sense of body awareness while exercising. As a result, it provides an

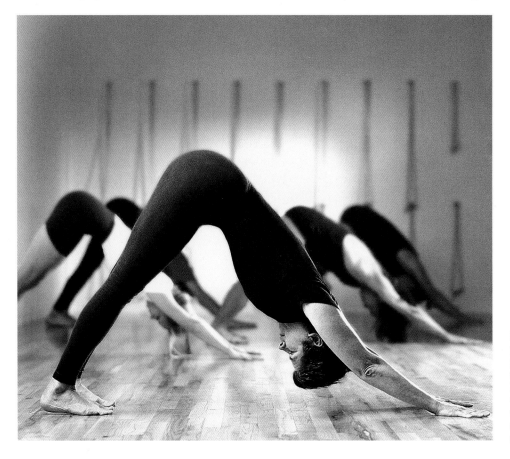

LEFT: **Regular yoga practice has a powerful effect in stimulating energy levels while also contributing to enhanced muscle stamina, strength and flexibility.**

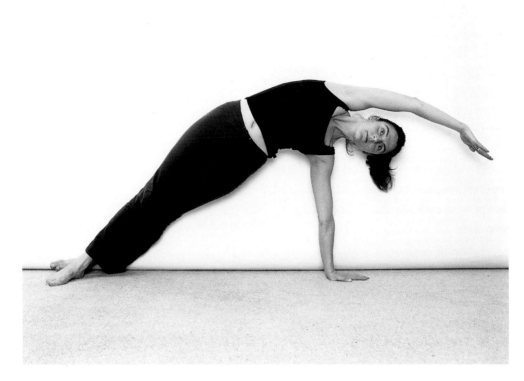

excellent contrast to the mindset of frenetic aerobics classes of the 1980s, in which movements would be repeated with scant attention paid to emerging pain that might signify injury or damage.

Because the basic Pilates technique is tailored as much as possible to the requirements of the individual, a Pilates teacher should never force a pupil into a posture or exercise that feels inappropriate or uncomfortable to them. Instead, successful use of the Pilates method involves learning how to perform precise muscular movements for a strictly limited number of repetitions. In other words, the main emphasis is put on accuracy of execution, rather than doing endless repetitions of exercises wrongly.

Once adept at Pilates, people find that their muscles appear longer and leaner as their posture becomes more aligned. In addition, regular practice should result in weak muscles being strengthened, and tense, tight muscles being stretched and relaxed.

T'ai Chi

T'ai chi is an excellent system of movement to consider if you feel you need extra help in promoting muscular flexibility and enhanced co-ordination. It is also an invaluable tool to use to promote a positive state of harmony of mind and body. The practice of t'ai chi involves the execution of graceful, slow movements that are co-ordinated with breathing techniques. When this technique is mastered, the overall effect should be one of a general sense of well-being, a profound feeling of calm, and increased physical and emotional resilience.

In common with yoga, which also lays great emphasis on the importance of proper breathing technique to promote an energizing or relaxing effect, t'ai chi stimulates a balanced and healthy flow of energy (called "qi" – pronounced "chee") throughout the body. It has a great deal in common with the Chinese healing system, acupuncture, which also seeks to stimulate the healthy flow of qi along the meridians – unseen channels of energy that the Chinese believe traverse the body – through the insertion of fine acupuncture needles at specific points on these invisible channels.

Claims have been made that t'ai chi can promote mental and emotional clarity, improve general flexibility, encourage relaxation of the muscles and nervous system, and help maintain the efficiency of breathing patterns without the drawback of putting extra strain on the heart.

Qi Gong

Qi gong (pronounced "chee gong") has similar aims to t'ai chi and conveys parallel benefits. It is a system of meditation in movement that seeks to stimulate the balanced flow of energy (qi) through the body. Thus, it can be regarded as a system of physical movement that fits well within the context of tradi-

tional Chinese medicine, with its core concern of promoting the balanced and enhanced flow of qi energy.

As an extension of this idea, qi gong embraces the need for stimulating optimum balance and harmony on emotional, mental, and physical levels while also developing a keen sense of body awareness. Once followers have become familiar with regular practice of qi gong, they find they reach a point where energy levels are optimally balanced, while mind and emotions should also feel harmonized and relaxed.

In qi gong, specific parts of the body are endowed with a particular significance and importance. These include the

BELOW: **The graceful, fluid movements of t'ai chi are thought to have a profoundly relaxing effect on mind and body, producing mental and emotional clarity.**

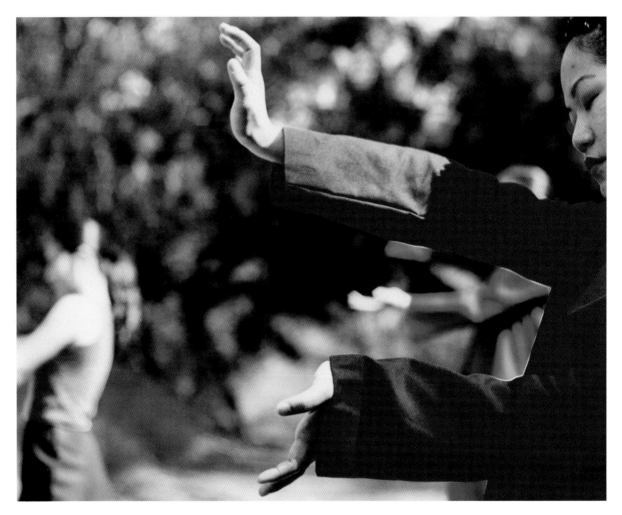

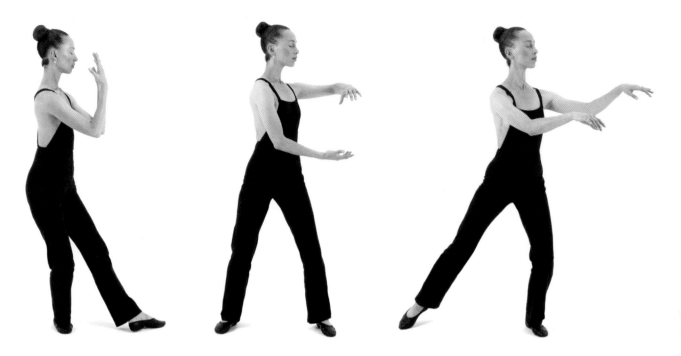

ABOVE: **Qi gong, like acupuncture and acupressure, is concerned with stimulating the optimum flow of energy through the body.**

crown of the head, the forehead, tongue, navel, perineum, the palms of the hands and the soles of the feet. By developing a consciousness of these specific areas and breathing in a conscious and controlled way, it is thought that mental, emotional and physical balance, equilibrium, and vitality can all be enhanced.

Alexander Technique

Although not strictly speaking an exercise technique, the Alexander technique has a place in any discussion of the merits and advantages of physical fitness and its effects on the mind and body.

The Alexander Technique concentrates on teaching how posture can affect emotional experience and vice-versa. This can be of particular value in any situation where you feel tense and stressed as learning the basics of the technique can set those practising the technique free from patterns of mental and emotional behaviour that may have become ingrained and established.

The Alexander Technique helps break physical and mental habits that may feel like second nature, because they have become so familiar. This is done by teaching an awareness of the physical reactions that occur when people are placed in a threatening or excessively stressful situation. Once you recognize the physical habits you have developed in response to these unsettling stimuli, you are empowered to make a conscious choice as to whether you want to continue to react in this way, or not.

Becoming familiar with the Alexander Technique can be an excellent starting point from which to explore any exercise system that demands a strong sense of body awareness. By developing such body awareness through the Alexander Technique, you are unlikely to bring poor postural habits to whatever exercise system you have chosen to undertake. Indeed, you are much more likely to derive maximum benefit from it, especially if it involves very precise movements of specific muscle groups, such as those used in Pilates.

Body-Conditioning Treats

Now that we have considered ways of enhancing optimum functioning of the immune system from within (by stimulating enhanced lymphatic drainage through exercise systems that encourage regular, rhythmic muscle movements, or by techniques that de-stress the mind), we can look at ways of stimulating more efficient flow of lymphatic fluid from without.

Both the techniques described in this section are based on a loosely naturopathic approach, with the emphasis on straightforward measures that can easily be followed at home. They will not take ages to do, nor do they require special, expensive equipment and knowledge to accomplish. Most important of all, they are likely to make you feel energized, vibrant and full of vitality, while also promoting significant cosmetic advantages in the form of smoother skin tone and texture.

Dry-skin Brushing

This is one of the simplest methods of encouraging effective detoxing of the system through stimulation of drainage of lymphatic fluid. All that is needed to start is a natural bristle brush, ideally with a long handle so that it can treat hard-to-reach areas of the body. Here's how to do it:

- Get into the habit of spending a few minutes dry-skin brushing before taking a bath or shower.
- Brush in large, sweeping movements that cover your body, moving upwards from the feet and legs to the hips on the front and back, while also brushing in a downward movement to the trunk.
- Keep the pressure steady, but not so heavy that it causes any discomfort.
- Always avoid brushing any areas of irritated, inflamed or broken skin or patches where poor circulation has led to the appearance of broken or thread veins.
- After covering the body with smooth, invigorating strokes on the dry skin, cleanse the skin surface by taking a stimulating shower or soaking in a warm (but not too hot) and soothing bath.

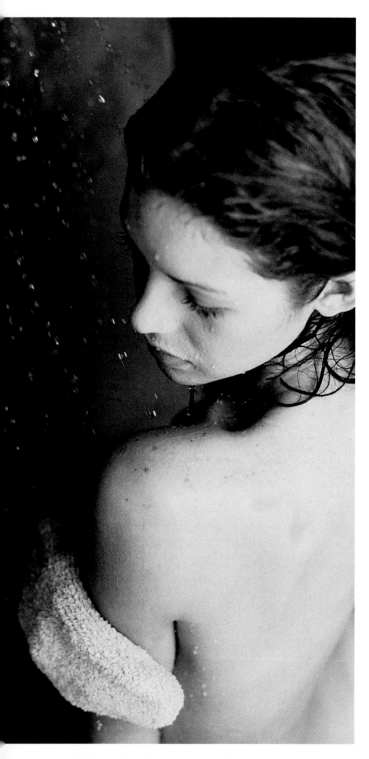

ABOVE: **Using a body scrub regularly in the shower keeps the skin smooth and receptive to the body products that follow.**

Simple Hydrotherapy Techniques

Water is essential to life: we can survive for a surprisingly long period of time without food, but we can become life-threateningly dehydrated very rapidly. This is particularly the case with illnesses that very quickly deplete the body of fluid, especially in the very young or the elderly. The body is made up of approximately 70 per cent liquid, and is fundamentally dependent on the circulation of this liquid to maintain the smooth and efficient maintenance of basic body functions.

Not only does water play a central role in ensuring our physical survival in this way, but it can also give us a sense of emotional and physical well-being and vitality when used in the form of hydrotherapy.

The benefits that may be conveyed through the use of simple, practical hydrotherapy techniques include:
- improved skin appearance, tone and texture
- greater vitality
- enhanced protection against recurrent minor illnesses

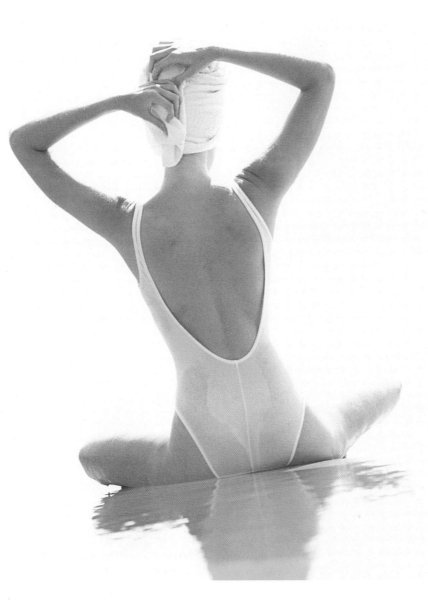

LEFT: **Regular use of hydrotherapy techniques can have a revitalizing effect on the mind and body.**

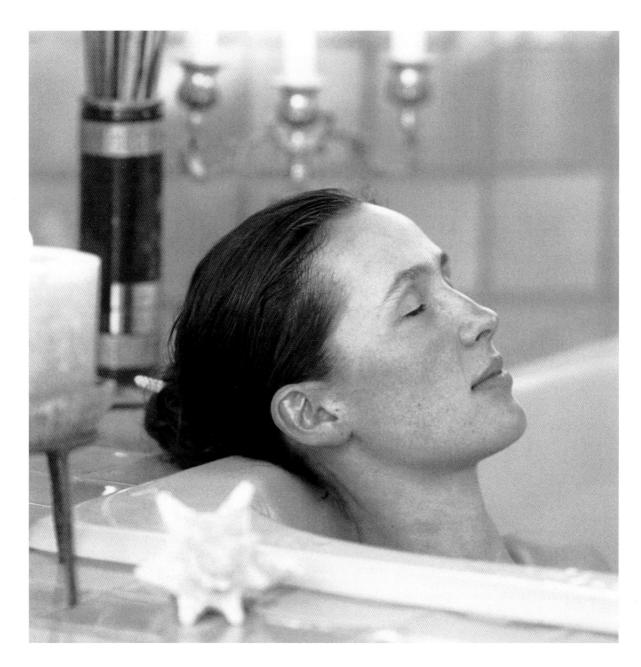

ABOVE: **The ideal temperature for bath water is comfortably warm rather than too hot. Excessively hot water can have an adverse effect on skin tone and texture and cause it to sag.**

- fewer skin problems and conditions
- reduction in catarrhal and congestive problems as toxins are eliminated more effectively through the skin
- improved circulation

- enhanced function of eliminatory organs such as the kidneys, bowel and lungs

Provided you are generally in good health with no problems such as heart disease, angina, varicose veins or ulcers, chronic skin problems such as eczema or psoriasis or high blood pressure, the hydrotherapy techniques described here may do may do a great deal to banish sluggishness and stimulate a renewed sense of vitality. If you are in any doubt as to the advisability of pursuing these techniques because of concerns about being unfit, always consult your doctor before embarking on any course of action.

Here are the main points to consider when giving yourself hydrotherapy treatment at home:

- Hydrotherapy treatments given at European spa resorts use extremely high-power water jets directed at specific parts of the body to stimulate enhanced circulation. You can achieve a less drastic version by using a hand-held domestic shower.
- Start by taking a moderately warm shower until comfortable. Once you are ready to begin treatment, switch to the cold setting for approximately twenty seconds, before moving back to warm again. If you feel able, finish off with another burst of cold. If you feel uneasy at first with as much as twenty seconds' exposure to cold water, only take as much as you feel at ease with, building up slowly. Also bear in mind that it is possible to have too much of a good thing, and that you should never aim to go beyond a maximum of thirty seconds' exposure to a cold shower.
- It is extremely important to make sure that you never start with a cold shower when you feel generally chilled and uncomfortable. Make a deliberate point of warming up first, either by some gentle exercise, or by having a comfortably warm shower.
- If you want to aim for a more stimulating, directed, vitality-inducing effect, direct the shower head down the body, moving from the head and face, down the arms, belly and legs.
- If you feel specific areas need attention to tone up tissues that are showing the negative effects of gravity (such as the breasts), these areas can be targeted with a spray of cold water.
- Once a hydrotherapy session is over, it is helpful to leave damp areas that are to be covered by clothing to dry naturally, rather than vigorously towel-drying the whole body. It is generally beneficial to stay in a warm temperature until thoroughly dry, to avoid becoming chilled.
- Bathing can also be a very valuable way of exploiting the therapeutic powers of water, provided certain rules are borne in mind. These include avoiding the use of water that is too hot because this can have a negative effect on skin tone, causing it to sag and become excessively dehydrated. Extended hot baths can also lead you to feel unpleasantly enervated rather than energized or pleasantly relaxed.
- You can make bath-time a relaxing, soothing experience or an invigorating, energizing pick-me-up, depending on what you choose to add to the bath water. Essential oils can have a powerful effect on the mind and emotions: use a few drops of oils with invigorating or unwinding properties as you choose. If you prefer not to soak in oil-scented, warm water, have an essential-oil diffuser near at hand, or a candle scented with essential oils burning in the bathroom. Stimulating essential oils include rosemary, peppermint, bergamot, coriander and grapefruit. Relaxing essential oils include chamomile, rose, lavender and ylang ylang.
- Enhance the detoxing effects of bathing by indulging in a powdered seaweed or natural mud treatment. The former can be dissolved in the bath water and the latter can be applied to the body and showered off before bathing. When taking a detoxing seaweed bath, always avoid soaking in hot water which will make the bath tension-making and exhausting rather than an aid to detox. After soaking in a warm bath (approximately body heat), shower off any residue of the seaweed mixture before wrapping up cosily in a towel wrap and taking it easy for an hour or so. It also helps to drink plenty of still mineral water after a treatment of this kind to support the body's eliminative processes.

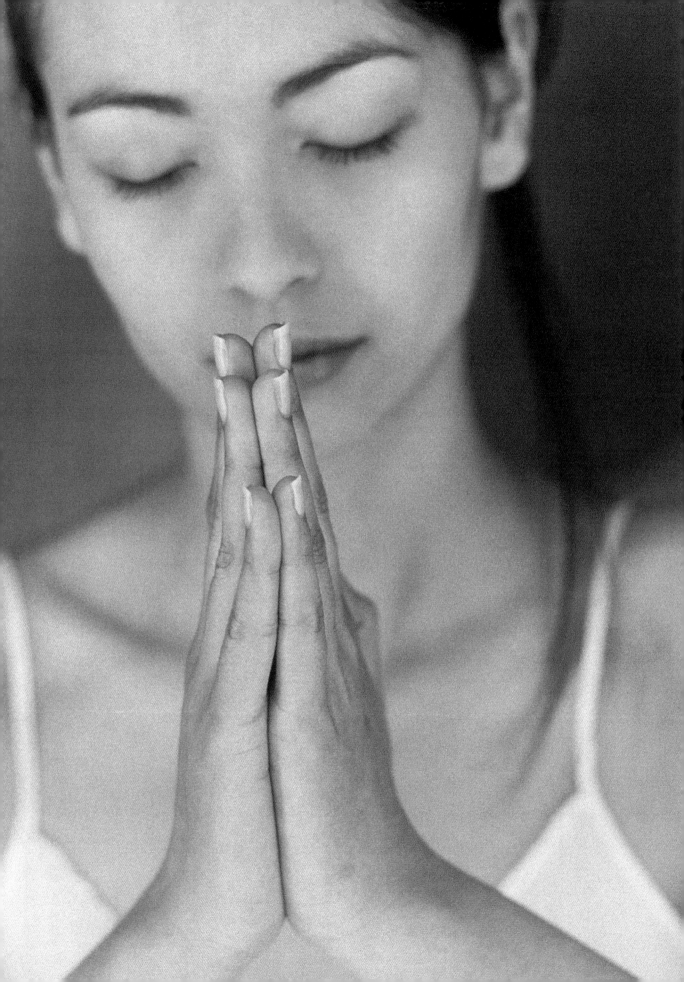

Strange as it may sound, we really can think ourselves well. As we have already seen in Chapter 2 specific links have been made between the onset of protracted distressing or stressful experiences and the development or deterioration of stress-related illnesses such as high blood pressure, irritable bowel syndrome and degenerative heart disease.

What is of even greater interest is the revelation that negative emotional experiences appear to have a direct effect on the performance of the immune system. This has been demonstrated through the work of Dr Simonton in the United States, who has had good results using positive visualization techniques with cancer patients, and by some recent British studies that have explored the physiological impact of pleasurable or uplifting thoughts.

The British studies include one recently carried out at the University of Reading, which demonstrated that participants who positively recalled pleasurable thoughts and memories had increased levels of immune antibodies on analysis of saliva samples, taken before and after the memories were evoked. Those participants in the study who had dwelt on distressing or stressful thoughts were shown to have depressed levels of immune antibodies.

It has been suggested that sensual influences can also play some part in affecting the body's defences. Research carried out by Associates for Research into the Science of Enjoyment (ARISE) revealed that the immune system may

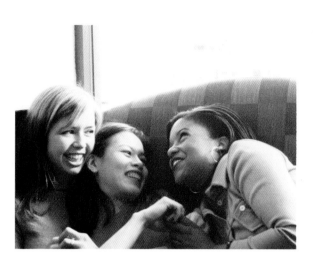

ABOVE: **It's a fact: laughter is good for the immune system, providing an outlet for reducing stress hormones.**

respond positively or negatively to sensual impressions, depending on whether they are pleasurable or repellent in nature. During the course of the study it was found that levels of the immune system antibody SIgA measured in saliva samples were affected in a favourable or destructive way, as the subjects were exposed to a range of attractive or unpleasant odours such as chocolate or rotten meat. Researchers concluded that exposure to pleasure-giving sensual impressions can boost immune- system performance, while contact with unpleasant odours can do the reverse.

Other research studies have shown that how much we laugh may also have an impact on the performance of our

7 Boosting Immunity
with Relaxation

immune systems. The positive effect of a good chortle is thought to be connected to the way in which laughter may perform an important outlet in reducing stress hormones. Sex is another release that may play a big part in bolstering the body's defences, as well as giving us sensual pleasure. It has been revealed that people who have sex at least twice a week have higher circulating levels of IgA antibodies than those who abstain from sex, or who enjoy a less than lively sex life.

Stress and the Immune System

There appears to be strong links between the amount of stress we are exposed to, the way in which we deal with this strain, and our immune systems. Stress is a fact of life for most people and few of us are likely to enjoy a stress-free daily experience of life. We can learn to identify how much negative stress there is in our lives and observe how we react to such stress. We are then free to explore stress-reducing and stress-managing techniques that will help us live life to the full and in a balanced way.

Before examining these issues more closely, it will help to understand first how and why stress has an impact on the way the immune system performs.

Fight or Flight?

When we react to an overly-stressful situation, a number of physiological changes, called the "fight or flight response", take place. Our blood pressure rises, extra blood is circulated to our extremities to prepare us to run from physical danger, and our digestive organs register a change in pattern of function that may make us feel queasy or make us want to empty our bowels quickly. All of these changes are designed to prepare us for a rapid physical response to a threatening situation. Unfortunately, most of the stressful situations we are likely to encounter on a day-to-day basis can't be sprinted away from, but have to be solved by another route.

Certain hormonal changes also take place as part of a stress response, with stress hormones such as adrenaline and cortisol rising rapidly. Blood sugar levels are also affected,

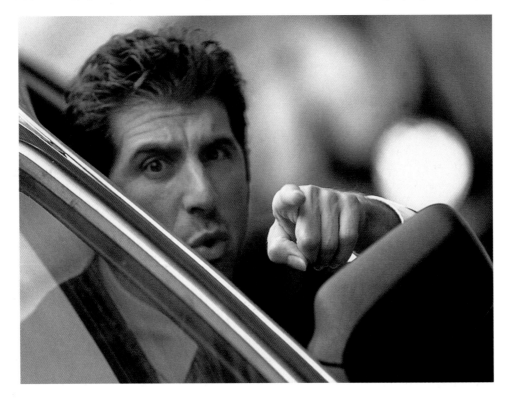

LEFT: **Unresolved, mounting stress levels, such as are often experienced by motorists, can contribute to compromised immune-system performance.**

rising to provide us with extra energy to accomplish whatever response is needed. If we are in a situation where we are able to channel our energies into a physical response, such as sprinting away from or fighting a physical threat, we should find that our bodies can relax once the danger is over, and reach a state of equilibrium once again.

Things are very different if we are experiencing these physiological changes on a frequent basis in an inappropriate situation, which could include anything from being confronted with an unexpectedly large bill to arguing with our partner or having a work-load or financial pressure that we feel powerless to meet.

If this negative pattern goes on for a long period without our discovering effective tools to enable us to manage stress and to relax, we are very likely to experience unwelcome stress-related problems. These may include high blood pressure, stress-related headaches, migraines, stomach ulcers, irritable bowel syndrome, insomnia, palpitations and numerous other conditions.

In addition, there are subtler links between our state of mind and emotions and the functioning of the immune system that can give rise to recurrent minor infections, allergies, and auto-immune disorders, such as rheumatoid arthritis and cancer. The burgeoning science of psycho-neuroimmunology has also drawn attention to the way in which powerful emotions and a generally optimistic or pessimistic outlook can affect immune-system functioning.

We should, we are told, regard our nervous and immune systems as being intimately interlinked. Neuropeptides (the chemical messengers that communicate with the hormonal, nervous and immune systems) appear to be measurably affected positively or negatively by emotional reactions. In addition, our immune-system cells have receptors for the stress hormones adrenaline and noradrenaline, secretions that are directly implicated in the fight or flight response. As a result, ongoing, unresolved negative stress is likely to have a perceptible effect on the body's defences.

It appears that unmanaged, excessive negative stress is one of the major triggers for putting an excessive amount of strain on the immune system. We should make stress

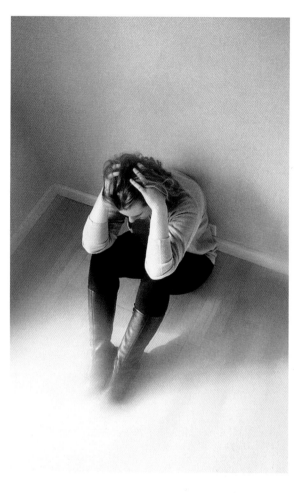

ABOVE: **Depression is an immensely cruel illness that can make us feel stressed, lonely and unable to cope.**

management techniques a priority if we live pressured lives and want to boost our body's basic capacity for self- healing.

Negative and Positive Stress

Before moving on to learning some basic techniques for banishing unhealthy levels of pressure and inducing a more balanced, relaxed state of emotions, mind, and body, it is important to explore the basic nature of stress so that we can differentiate between its positive and negative aspects.

We hear so much about stress-related problems that it may come as a shock to learn that some forms of stress can be beneficial. If life were to become totally stress-free, we could become sluggish, lacking in motivation and bored. If we have

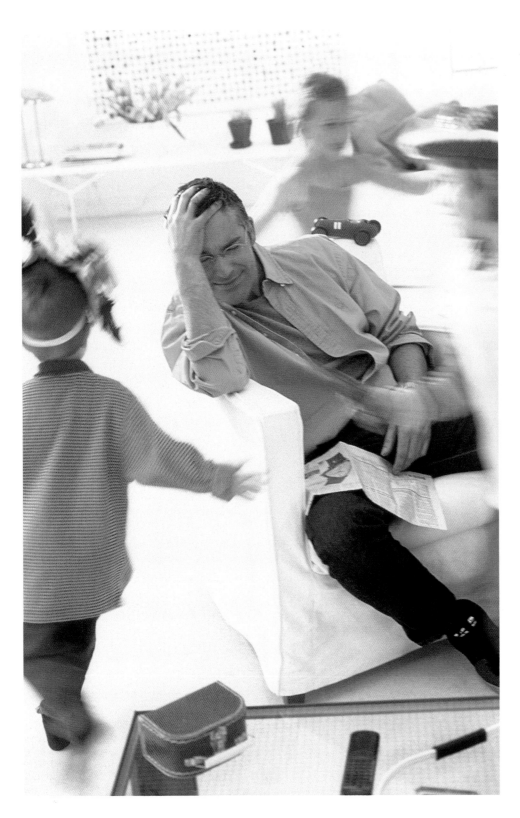

CHAPTER 7

LEFT: Negative stress occurs when people feel unable to cope with the pressures around them, such as when demanding days at work are regularly followed by encountering lively children with demands of their own at home.

enough positive stress in our lives to provide challenges we know we can meet if we make an extra effort, this can be an important ally in helping us feel focused, alert and satisfied. The key to making the most of positive stress in our lives is to achieve a state of balance. We should not feel overwhelmed by the demands made on us; rather, we should be stimulated by them. When this basic balance exists, we should find that the sense of achievable pressure exerted on us gives us just enough extra adrenaline to give us the mental or physical "edge" we need to achieve whatever challenge has been set us. After this has been met, we should feel relaxed, especially if we draw on some of the techniques listed below to speed up the relaxation and recovery process.

Feeling powerless in the face of the demands made on us, and being unable to act to resolve whatever situation we have been presented with, can lead to a cycle of negative stress. If this occurs, we are likely to feel both indecisive and confused, rather than feeling clear-headed and ready to be spurred to constructive action. Being faced with a presentation or examination that we have not been able to prepare for adequately is a good example of the kind of situation that can cause negative stress. Positive stress, on the other hand, could arise from being well-prepared to face the examination, so that we feel in control of ourselves and of the situation.

Basic Techniques for De-stressing and Relaxation

Stress does not inevitably have to be a problem. It is the nature of the way in which we deal with it – the techniques we employ – that is of paramount importance when it comes to dealing with stress. Here, we look at the several techniques that may be employed.

Relaxation Techniques

If we are overloaded with negative stress it can be infuriating to be told to "just relax". For those who are naturally laid-back, "relaxing" is not a problem. Those who suffer from feeling tense and anxious need to learn how to begin to unwind, since it is not something that is second nature to them. There are a number of helpful routes open to developing a practical strategy for relaxing.

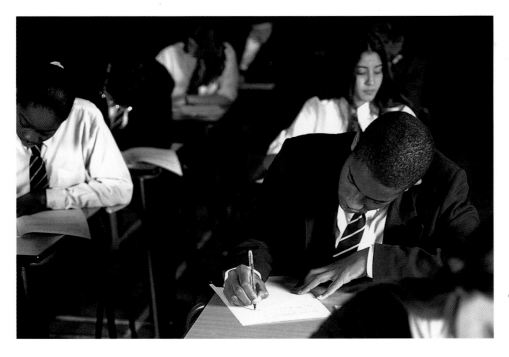

LEFT: **Positive stress involves feeling challenged, stimulated and in a position to cope effectively with pressure.**

For those who prefer to be taught in a group setting, attending a well-taught yoga class could be the answer. This can give the double advantage of learning physical postures that can strengthen and condition the body and learning breathing techniques that can enable you to reach a profound sense of physical, mental and emotional relaxation. If you prefer to learn how to relax in private, there are plenty of audio cassettes and CDs available that will talk you through a guided relaxation exercise programme. Deciding on this approach has the advantage of flexibility, because you can choose the setting and time of day that suits you best for practising a relaxation technique.

Autogenic Training

This form of relaxation can be immensely helpful in enabling you to deal with feelings of on-going tension and anxiety. Getting to grips with the technique involves learning a number of specific mental exercises which suggest that certain sensations are being felt in the body. These suggestions are likely to include sensations of warmth, heaviness or lack of tension in specific areas of the body (for example, "my hand is getting warm and heavy").

Even though you are initially learning how to induce a

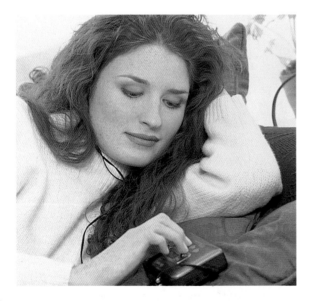

ABOVE: **Custom-made relaxation audio tapes can be an invaluable help in encouraging us to switch off and unwind.**

conscious state of relaxation in specific areas of the body, once you have mastered the technique, you should reach a point where functions of the body normally considered to be involuntary in nature (in other words, not under conscious control) also benefit. These could include reduced pulse or heart rate. When this occurs, you will be able to trigger a profound sense of relaxation within a comparatively rapid time scale.

Autogenic training is very appealing in its simplicity. You do not need any special paraphernalia or equipment to reap the benefits of the relaxation that it can bring. Provided you get into the habit of practising the technique on a regular basis, you should find that you develop the necessary skills of physical observation that allow you to become familiar with what a sense of deep relaxation feels like.

To learn the technique, it is best to seek teaching from a trained therapist, rather than attempting to learn autogenic training by yourself. This is important because sometimes emotions surface as the technique is practised that the learner may find difficult to work through on his or her own. Access to an experienced practitioner means access to the necessary skills and training to evaluate and respond to any reactions that may surface.

Meditation

Meditation is an invaluable tool that can be drawn whenever you feel stressed and tense, and need to tune out mentally and emotionally. If you meditate every day, you are likely to reap the benefits of feeling emotionally, mentally and physically calmer, while also being able to bring greater clarity of mind and enhanced concentration to any mental tasks at hand.

ACHIEVING A MEDITATIVE STATE

- Make sure the room you are sitting in is as comfortably warm as possible so that you will not be unnecessarily distracted by feeling unduly cold or overheated.
- Sit in a straight-backed chair so that your spine is given maximum support.
- Focus gently on an image that you find attractive. This could be a flower or a candle that is sitting in front of

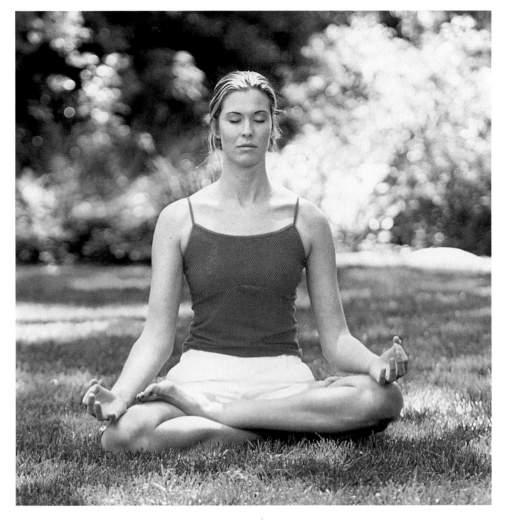

you at eye level, or it could be a simple image generated in your mind that you can call up with your eyes closed.

- If you feel that you can work more effectively with a verbal sound than a visual image, you can repeat out loud a single syllable over and over to yourself.
- Try to empty your conscious mind of any worrying or distracting thoughts, and gaze at your image or repeat your sound to yourself as you focus on your breathing, which should be regular and smooth in pattern.

Don't worry if distracting thoughts push themselves into your mind. This is very likely to happen at first. Just try gently to put them to one side and continue with your meditation exercise. The main thing to remember about meditation is that it needs to be made part of your daily routine if you are to reap the maximum de-stressing benefits that it can bring.

Creative Visualization Techniques

Positive visualization can be used as an effective part of a relaxation session. You need to be in a warm, comfortable, peaceful and relaxed environment. Once you feel fully unwound, you should close your eyes and in your mind's eye picture a place you find especially tranquil or attractive. This scene can be as detailed or as incomplete as you choose to make it. You should then move on to imagining yourself within the setting you have pictured to yourself, taking pleasure in all the sensual

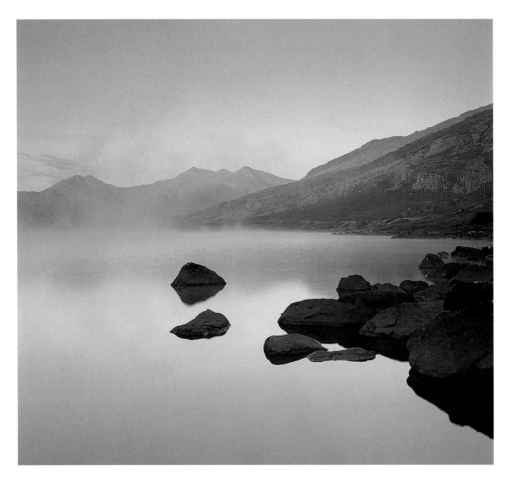

impressions surrounding you. You can remain in this place for as long as you feel you need to. When you open your eyes, you should feel calm, peaceful and refreshed.

Alternatively, you can imagine yourself being filled from head to foot with a liquid that symbolizes a sense of well-being, tranquillity and calm. When you feel fully relaxed, you can picture the same liquid leaving your body from top to toe, with a lasting sense of well-being and emotional and mental balance being left behind.

Basic Breathing Techniques

How we breathe has a direct effect on how we feel, especially if we are tense and anxious. By developing a sense of how we can breathe to induce a sense of relaxation and calm, we are giving ourselves an important anxiety-diffusing boost. The reason for this is quite simple. When we are fearful and uptight, we tend to breathe rapidly and in a shallow way from our upper chests. If we learn how to breathe with our maximum lung capacity in an unforced and rhythmical way, we are balancing the ratio between oxygen and carbon dioxide in our systems. As we do this, we should begin to feel calmer, more relaxed, and clear-headed.

If you hyperventilate – that is, breathe quickly from the upper chest – because of anxiety, you get in a vicious circle where you feel more up-tight and panicky due to an imbalance between carbon dioxide and oxygen in the bloodstream, which contributes to an ever-increasing sense of anxiety, which makes you even more inclined to hyperventilate. If this goes on long enough, you can feel yourself spiralling into a state of chronic stress in which panic attacks may occur.

This trend can be reversed extremely effectively, as soon as you become familiar with the practical tools of relaxed

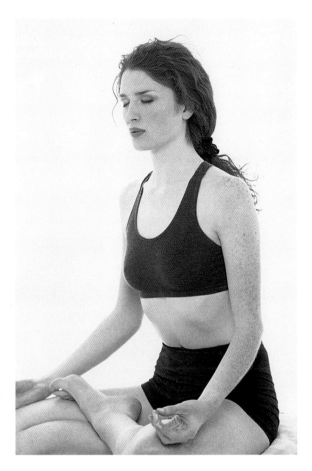

ABOVE: **Concentrating on breathing techniques can induce a sense of mental, emotional and physical well-being.**

breathing techniques. Once you get the hang of the basic idea, it is a wonderfully simple and effective way to induce a peaceful and calm state of mind and body.

To breathe with maximum lung capacity, you need to breath from your diaphragm, a sheet of muscle that lies at the bottom of the ribs and lungs. To locate where this is, rest one hand on the abdomen at roughly the level of your navel. As you breathe in fully, you should find that the belly rises and pushes your hand up and outwards. As you breathe out, your hand should sink back in to its original position. Once you have become used to this sensation, you should take a deep, slow breath in, making sure that your full lung capacity is being brought into play. As you gently breathe out fully, you should find that your lungs are emptying from the base to the tip.

If you take a few breaths in this way, making sure that you keep the rhythm steady, slow, and even, you should find that you begin to feel calmer and more clear-headed within a comparatively short space of time. If there is any sensation of dizziness or wooziness, you can rectify the problem by breathing normally for a moment or two until you feel back to normal. Then you can start diaphragmatic breathing once again.

Once you are familiar with the sensations involved, you will no longer need to rest your hand on your belly to achieve a fully relaxing breathing technique. As a result, you will be able to call on this important, stress-relieving tool wherever and whenever you feel under pressure.

Positive Thinking

Since thinking positively appears to have an immune system-boosting effect, you should make a particular effort to replace habitual negative thought patterns with more positive thoughts.

In the same way that you can adopt a physical postural habit that has a negative effect on the body (such as tension in the neck and shoulders leading to recurrent headaches and back pain), you can fall into the habit of negative thought patterns without consciously realizing it. These can feel so natural that you may not even consider that you have a choice in looking at situations from a more positive perspective. If you feel you have a particularly well-established problem like this, you should consider seeking help from a cognitive therapist who is trained to show people how to break negative patterns that may have been set up as far back as childhood.

OVERCOMING A TEMPORARILY NEGATIVE PERSPECTIVE

If you feel that, generally, you are pretty optimistic, but that, faced with an unexpected pressure or crisis, you tend to take on a view of things that is temporarily negative, the following suggestions may help you overcome the problem.

- Try to be less hard on yourself if you have a tendency to blame yourself unjustly for everything that may go wrong. A basic ability to take responsibility is essential to leading a balanced adult life, but heaping blame on yourself where it is not merited can be a sign of a lack of self-esteem.

- Appreciate your strengths and start to like yourself. The latter can be one of the hardest things to do if you are not encouraged to value your own gifts and strong points.
- When in emotional pain, don't suppress it and keep a stiff upper lip, but allow yourself to grieve in your own natural way and at your own individually-dictated pace. This can apply to a whole range of life experiences including bereavement, the break-up of a relationship, the loss of a valued job, or a change in personal identity through getting older.
- Be aware of negative emotions such as unreasonable anger, envy or resentment. These can be especially draining of vitality and need to be dealt with rather than allowed to fester and take root.
- If you feel that you are beginning to feel dominated by anxiety over a specific situation that is getting out of hand, try gaining a more reasonable perspective by picturing how important this particular anxiety-making episode is going to be in ten years time.

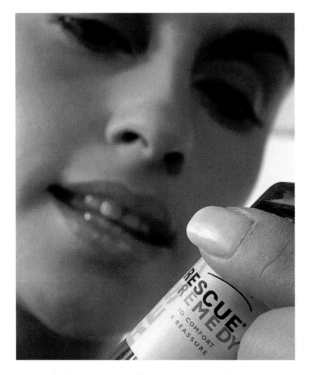

ABOVE: **Flower essences can be a practical aid to achieving emotional balance without side-effects.**

Alternative Hints for Relaxation

There are several alternative therapies that can offer considerable help in the matter of learning how to relax.

Herbal Help
An infusion of any of the following herbs can, when added to the bath water, induce a pleasant state of relaxation of body and mind:
- chamomile
- lavender
- rosemary
- lemon balm

Aromatherapy
A de-stressing effect may be obtained by adding a few drops of one of the following essential oils to the bath water, or vaporizing the oil in a custom-made diffuser:
- bergamot
- chamomile
- clary sage
- lavender
- ylang ylang

Bach Flower Remedies
Any of the following may be helpful where negative states of mind are a barrier to achieving a state of emotional equilibrium and relaxation:
- Pine may be indicated if stress is coming from a tendency to constantly take the blame for the mistakes of others.
- Beech is more suitable where there is a strong tendency to be a perfectionist, which leads to a lack of patience with the short-comings of others. As a result, emotional burn-out is combined with bursts of anger and extreme irritability.
- Elm may be indicated for classic burn-out symptoms, especially if there is a general tendency to take on an excessive workload, leading to feelings of being completely overwhelmed by responsibility.

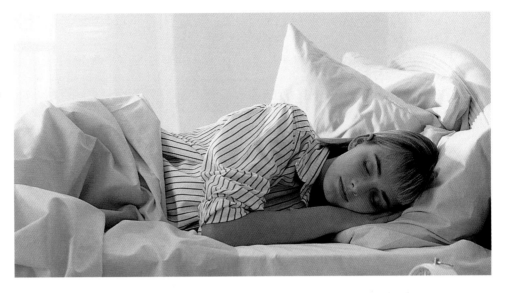

RIGHT: **Establishing a regular, refreshing sleep pattern is one of the most effective ways of maintaining mental, emotional and physical harmony.**

Homeopathic Support

ACONITE

Rapidly-descending feelings of anxiety and panic that are accompanied by palpitations and tremendous feelings of restlessness may be rapidly eased by Aconite.

GELSEMIUM

Tension and anxiety that is related to anticipation of a coming stressful event may respond to Gelsemium, if there is a general state of quiet preoccupation, weariness and trembling. In addition, there is likely to be a tension headache with a characteristic sensation of a tight band around the forehead and nervous, painless diarrhoea.

NUX VOMICA

A sensation of "burn-out" may respond to Nux vomica. Confirmatory symptoms for choice of this remedy include a tendency to rely on stimulants such as coffee to keep going, and alcohol and/or cigarettes to aid with unwinding. Characteristic features include poor sleep pattern and sleep quality, muscle tension, mental exhaustion, and digestive upsets.

Nutritional Hints

There are specific foods and drinks that should be avoided when you are feeling tense and under pressure, since they have a reputation for making things worse, not better. These are, paradoxically, the very same foods and drinks that many people tend to reach for when they feel pressured. They include:

- strong tea
- coffee
- sugary items
- alcohol
- chocolate

These all have a tendency to contribute to making you tense, jittery, and on a short fuse. In addition, food and drinks containing caffeine or alcohol can aggravate sleep problems, which can contribute further to compromised immune-system functioning.

There is no need to feel deprived, however, since there is a range of healthy substitutes for these foods that will encourage a sense of relaxation. These include:

- herbal or fruit-flavoured infusions
- grain-based coffee substitutes
- decaffeinated coffee (making sure you opt for a brand that has used a water-filtering process, rather than using chemical solvents to remove the caffeine)
- naturally fruit-flavoured, low-sugar, carbonated, non-alcoholic drinks with herbal extracts.

Resources

United Kingdom

General

*Council for Complementary
and Alternative Medicine*
Park House
206–208 Latimer Road
London W10 6RE
Tel: 020 873 50400

Regulatory and Advisory Bodies for Alternative and Complementary Therapies

British Acupuncture Council
Park House
206–208 Latimer Road
London W10 6RE
Tel: 020 873 50400

Aromatherapy Organisations Council
PO Box 19834
London SE25 6WF
Tel: 020 8251 7912

British Autogenic Society
Royal London Homeopathic Hospital
Great Ormond Street
London WC1M 3HR
Tel: 020 7713 6336

British Chiropractic Association
Blagrave House
17 Blagrave Street
Reading
Berkshire RG1 1QB
Tel: 0118 950 5950

The Society of Homeopaths
2 Artizan Road
Northampton NN1 4HU
Tel: 01604 621 400

*Massage Therapy
Institute of Great Britain*
PO Box 2726
London NW2 4NR
Tel: 020 8208 1639

Osteopathic Information Service
PO Box 2704
Reading, Berkshire RG1 4YR
Tel: 01491 875 255

*British Society for Allergy,
Environmental and
Nutritional Medicine*
PO Box 28, Totten
Southampton SO40 2ZA

*National Institute
of Medical Herbalists*
56 Longbrook Street
Exeter, Devon EX4 6AH
Tel: 01392 426 022

Exercise Systems

British Wheel of Yoga
1 Hamilton Place
Boston Road
Sleaford
Lincolnshire, NG34 7ES
Tel: 01529 306 851

T'ai Chi Union of Great Britain
94 Felsham Road
London SW15 1DQ
Tel: 020 8780 1063

*Society of Teachers
of the Alexander Technique*
20 London House
266 Fulham Road
London SW10 9EL
Tel: 020 7351 9838

The Pilates Foundation
80 Camden Road
London E17 7NF
Tel: 07071 781 859

Supplements

The Nutri Centre
The Hale Clinic
7 Park Crescent
London W1N 3HE
Tel: 020 7436 5122

Australia

*Association of Traditional Health
Practicioners Incorporated*
PO Box 346
Elizabeth, South Australia 5112
Tel: 08 8284 2324

United States

American Association of Acupuncture
and Oriental Medicine
4101 Lake Boone Trail Suite 201
Raleigh, North Carolina 27607
Tel: 919 787 5181

American Aromatherapy Association
PO Box 3679
South Pasadena, California 91031
Tel: 818 457 1742

American Chiropractic Association
1701 Clarendon Blvd
Arlington, Virginia 22209
Tel: 703 276 8800

American Herbalist Guild
PO Box 1683
Soquel, California 95073

National Centre for Homeopathy
801 North Fairfax Street, Suite 306
Alexandria, Virginia 22314
Tel: 703 548 7790

International Association of Yoga
Therapists
109 Hillside Avenue
Mill Valley, California 94941
Tel: 415 383 4587

Canada

Acupuncture Canada
107 Leitch Drive, Grimsby
Ontario, L3M 2T9
Tel: 1 905 563 9830

The Canadian Herb Society
5251 Oak Street
Vancouver
British Columbia V6M 4H1

Tzu Chi Institute
for Complementary Medicine
715 West 12th Avenue, Health Centre
4th Floor West, Vancouver
British Columbia, V4Z 1M9
Tel: 604 875 4769

Recommended Reading

Corbett, Nancy, *Boosting Your Immune System:
Help Prevent the Effects of Today's Health Problems
and Recover Vitality*, Sally Milner Publishing, 1991

Dr Sarah Brewer, *The Total Detox Plan:
A Comprehensive Programme to Cleanse Your
Mind and Body*, Carlton Books, 2000

Holford, Patrick, *One Hundred Percent Health:
The Drug Free Guide to Feeling Better, Living Longer
and Staying Free from Disease*, Piatkus, 1998

Kenton, Leslie, *Cellulite Revolution: Six Steps
to a New Body Ecology*, Random House, 1992

Kenton, Leslie, *Nature's Child: Guide, Nourish and
Protect Your Child the Gentle Way*, Random House, 1993

Levy, Elinor and Monte, Tom, *The Ten Best Tools
to Boost Your Immune System, A Total Health Prescription*,
Houghton Mifflin, 1997

MacEoin, *Come Alive: Your Six Point Plan for Lasting
Health and Energy*, Hodder and Stoughton, 2000

MacEoin, Beth, *Natural Medicine; A Practical
Guide to Family Health*, Bloomsbury, 1999

Vanderhaeghe, Lorna and Bouic, Patrick, *The Immune
System Cure: Optimize Your Immune System in Thirty
Days – The Natural Way*, Kensington Publishing, 1999

Index

A

adaptive immune system 12–13, 31–3
acidophilus acid 88
aconite 70, 123
ageing 23
AIDS 20
alcohol 39
Alexander technique 107
allergies 17–19
aloe vera 93
alternative medicines 8–9, 13–14
antigens 13
antihistamines 18
antioxidants 55–65
aromatherapy 69, 77, 82, 84, 88, 93, 122
arsenicum album 82, 94
Associates for Research into the Science
    of Enjoyment 112
auto-immune disorders 20–1
autogenic training 118

B

B-cells 14–16, 18
Bach flower remedies 122
barley 81
basil 69
belladonna 84–5
beta-carotene 58–60
body-conditioning 108–11
boiling 53
bone marrow 11–12, 14, 15
borax 89
Brazil nuts 62–3
breast-feeding 12
breathing techniques 120–1
bryonia 78
burn-out 71–5

C

cancer 20–1

cantharis 82
caprylic acid 88
carbo veg 94
cell-mediated response 18–19
cellulite 28
chamomile 81
chicken pox 13
citrus fruits 41
co-enzyme Q10 64
coffee 37
colds 67–70
coltsfoot 78
conventional medicines 16–7, 18, 31
cooking 51–3, 58, 61
coughs 75–8
cranberry juice 81
cruciferous vegetables 41–2
cystitis 79–82

D

dairy products 19
deep frying 52–3
dehydration 37
digestive upsets 90–5
diuretics 37
dry-skin brushing 108

E

echinacea 68
elderberry 69
emotions 21, 98–100
endorphins 100
exercise 28–31, 72, 97–107

F

fats 42, 44
fatty acids 42–3, 44
fibre 42
first-line immunity 12
flu 17

free radicals 38, 40, 56–7
fruit 37, 39–42, 50–1, 60–1

G

garlic 45, 68, 77, 87
gelsemium 70, 123
ginseng 74
grapefruit 93
grapes 41
green tea 44
grilling 52

H

health:
    antioxidants 55–65
    body-conditioning 108–11
    exercise 28–31, 72, 97–107
    hydrotherapy 30–1
    and immune system 7, 17–19, 23–5
    nutrition 27–8, 34–9, 46–50, 123
    relaxation 17, 71–2, 112–23
    smoking 28, 38
    stress 25–6, 31, 71–5, 114–17
hepar sulph 85
herbal teas 45, 81
herbs 45, 68–9, 75, 78, 81, 84, 88, 94,
    122
histamine 18
HIV 20
homeopathic remedies 69–70, 78, 82,
    84–5, 89–90, 94, 122
hormones 16
hydrotherapy 30–1, 109–11
hypersensitivities 17–19

I

IgE antibodies 18–19
immune system:
    adapative immune system 12–13
    allergies 17–19

antioxidants 55–65
auto-immune disorders 20–1
definition 11–14
exercise 98
first-line immunity 12
and health 7, 17–19, 23–5
hypersensitive 17–19
natural immunity 12
nutrition 27–8, 46–50, 123
passive immunity 12
psychoneuroimmunology 25–6
relaxation 112–23
response to invader 14–16
stress 25–6, 31, 71–5, 114–17
vaccination 13–14
Interleukin 1 16
ipecac 94

K
kali bich 78
kali carb 89

L
lachesis 85
liver 14
"long-life" foods 36–7
lycopene 41
lymphatic fluid 28, 31
lymphocytes 14–16

M
macrophages 15–16
measles 13
meditation 118–19
microwaving 53
milk 76
monosodium glutamate 36
Mount Sinai Hospital School of Medicine
   25
mushrooms 46

N
natrum mur 70, 89
natural immunity 12
nutrition 27–8, 34–9, 46–50, 123
nux vomica 70, 94, 123

O
olive oil 41

P
passive immunity 12
phosphorus 78
Pilates 104–5
pollution 7
positive thinking 212–2
probiotics 45–6
prostaglandins 43
proteins 37
psychoneuroimmunology 25–6
pulsatilla 70, 78, 89–90, 94

Q
qi gong 106–7

R
reservatrol 41
relaxation 17, 71–2, 112–23
roasting 52

S
schisandra 74–5
selenium 62–3
shallow frying 52
skin 14
smoking 28, 38
sore throats 82–5
spleen 11
staphisagria 82
steaming 52
stir-frying 52

stress 25–6, 31, 71–5, 114–17
sugar 37–8
supplements 68, 74–5, 77, 81, 84, 87–8,
   93

T
T-cells 14–16, 20, 21
t'ai chi 105–6
tea 37, 44
thrush 85–90
thymus gland 11, 14
tiredeness 17

U
University of Reading 26

V
vaccination 13–14
vegetable oils 43
vegetables 37, 39–42, 50–1
visualization techniques 119–20
vitamin A 58–60
vitamin B 36, 75
vitamin B6 64–5
vitamin C 41, 60–1, 68, 81, 84
vitamin E 36, 61–2

W
white blood cells 15–16
wholewheat foods 35–6

Y
yoga 104
yoghurt 45–6

Z
zinc 63–4

Author's Acknowledgements

I would like to thank the following for their professionalism, practical help, and support during the writing of this book. First and foremost, my warmest thanks are due to my agent Teresa Chris who played a vitally important role at the outset of this project in her perpetually delightful, patient and good humoured way. Sarah Larter and the publishing team at Carlton also receive my appreciation for having executed the publishing of this book so speedily, efficiently and with an impressive vision and commitment. Dr Anand and Dr Anthea Anand also played their part in giving so willingly of their time and expertise in constructively commenting on the sections dealing with orthodox medical theory. Finally, but most important of all, my deepest thanks go to my husband Denis. He is always prepared to give the most practical support in discussing ideas in their early stages, giving proofs a last "once over" with his constantly eagle eye and keeping everything in perspective with his infectious, unfailing sense of humour.

Picture Credits

The publishers would like to thank the following sources for their kind permission to reproduce the pictures in this book:

The Anthony Blake Photo Library: 46 b/Martin Brigdale/52/53/Chris Seddon/57tr Matthew May/62r Maximillian; Carlton Books: Graham Atkins-Hughes 41 t / Mary Atkinson 14 b, 26,/S. Price & R. Truscott 37 t / Howard Shooter 1, 2, 3, 4, 18/19, 36 b, 34, 40 b, 43 t, 44 b, 47t; Reproduced by kind permission of the Pilates Foundation ® UK Ltd/Photographer Polly Borland 105; Corbis: Tony Arruza 93 / Ric Ergenbright 45 t / Layne Kennedy 5, 66; Image Bank: S. Achernar 98 / Color Day 21b, 28t, 115 / Paulo Curto 109 / Diggin/M.Loco 63t / Britt Erlanson 12 b, 79, 112, 116 / LD Gordon 119 / Ross M. Horowitz 42t, 74, / Will Hui 19 r /Anthony Johnson 60t / Frederic Jorez 70 /John P. Kelly 72 / Tom King 29 / Carol Kohen 24b / Pat Lacroix 76br /Romilly Lockyer 96, 99tl / David de Lossy 24 t / Regine M. 91 / Rita Maas 41r, 64b, 68, 77, 81, 88b, 95 / Marc Romanelli 82, 101, 110 /Juan Silva 108 / Anselm Spring 88t / James Stirling 25b/Andrew Unangst 8 / Steve Wrubel 48b / White Packert 16 b, 57tl / L. Wallach, Inc 38l / Guang Hui Xie 9 / Yellow Dog Prods. 114; Caroline Jones: 22, 78, 120; Retna: Jenny Acheson 118, 121 / Ken Kochey 83tl / Sandra Lousada 99b / Philip Reeson 90, 122; Science Photo Library:BSIP, MASO 67 / Oscar Burriel 10 / Eye of Science 13t, 20b / Don Fawcett 15b / Damien Lovegrove 33b / Dr. Gopal Murti 15t / NIBSC 14t; Getty Images Stone: 27t, 87br, 106, 107 / Elie Bernagern 56 l / 113 Peter Correz 1 / Pauline Cutler 117 / Jack Daniels 18l / Dale Durfee 6 / Laurence Dutton 39l / Chris Harvey 123 / Ian Logan 71 / Gerard Loucel 103 / Anthony Marsland 49t / Lori Adamski Peek 102 / Dave Rosenberg 104 / Joern Rynio 45b / Tom Stock 100 / Alan Thornton 76tl / Les Wies 32t

Every effort has been made to acknowledge correctly and contact the source and/copyright holder of each picture, and Carlton Books Limited apologises for any unintentional errors or omissions which will be corrected in future editions of this book.